Antenatal

For Elsevier
Content Strategist: Alison Taylor
Content Development Specialist: Veronika Watkins
Project Manager: Julie Taylor
Designer: Paula Catalano
Illustration Manager: Amy Faith Heyden

VOLUME **2**

MIDWIFERY ESSENTIALS

Antenatal

EDITION **2**

Helen Baston, BA(Hons), MMedSci, PhD, PGDipEd, ADM, RN, RM
Consultant Midwife Public Health;
Sheffield Teaching Hospitals NHS Foundation Trust, UK;
Honorary Researcher/Lecturer, University of Sheffield;
Honorary Lecturer Sheffield Hallam University, UK

Jenny Hall, EdD, MSc, RN, RM, ADM, PGDip(HE), SFHEA
Senior Midwifery Lecturer, Bournemouth University, UK

ELSEVIER

Edinburgh London New York Oxford Philadelphia St Louis Sydney Toronto

ELSEVIER

ISBN 978-0-7020-7098-3
e_ISBN 978-0-7020-7136-2

Notices
Practitioners and researchers must always rely on their own experience and knowledge in evaluating and using any information, methods, compounds or experiments described herein. Because of rapid advances in the medical sciences, in particular, independent verification of diagnoses and drug dosages should be made. To the fullest extent of the law, no responsibility is assumed by Elsevier, authors, editors or contributors for any injury and/or damage to persons or property as a matter of products liability, negligence or otherwise, or from any use or operation of any methods, products, instructions, or ideas contained in the material herein.

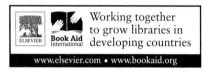

Working together
to grow libraries in
developing countries

www.elsevier.com • www.bookaid.org

your source for books,
journals and multimedia
in the health sciences

www.elsevierhealth.com

The
publisher's
policy is to use
**paper manufactured
from sustainable forests**

Printed in China

Contents

Preface

To contribute to the provision of sensitive, safe and effective maternity care for women and their families is a privilege. Childbirth is a life-changing event for women. Those around them and those who input into any aspect of pregnancy, labour, birth or the postnatal period can positively influence how this event is experienced and perceived. In order to achieve this, maternity carers continually need to reflect on the services they provide and strive to keep up to date with developments in clinical practice. They should endeavour to ensure that women are central to the decisions made and that real choices are offered and supported by skilled practitioners.

This book is the second volume in a series of texts based on the popular 'Midwifery Basics' series published in *The Practising Midwife* journal. The books have remained true to the original style of the articles and have been updated and expanded to create a user-friendly source of information. They are also intended to stimulate debate and require the reader both to reflect on their current practice, local policies and procedures and to challenge care that is not woman-centred. The use of scenarios enables the practitioner to understand the context of maternity care and explore their role in its safe and effective provision.

There are many dimensions to the provision of woman-centred care that practitioners need to consider and understand. To aid this process, a jigsaw model has been introduced, with the aim of encouraging the reader to explore maternity care from a wide range of perspectives. For example, how does a midwife obtain consent from a woman for a procedure, maintain a safe environment during the delivery of care and make the most of the opportunity to promote health? What are the professional and legal issues in relation to the procedure, and is this practice based on the best available evidence? Which members of the multi-professional team contribute to this aspect of care and how is it influenced by the way care is organized? Each aspect of the jigsaw should be considered during the assessment, planning, implementation and evaluation of woman-centred maternity care.

Midwifery Essentials: Antenatal (second edition) is about the provision of safe and effective care during pregnancy and preparation for birth. It reflects the focus of the National Maternity Review, *Better Births* (2016), endorsing personalized care and real choice for women. It comprises 10 chapters, each written to stand alone or be read in succession. The introductory chapter sets the scene, exploring the role of the midwife in the context of professional and national guidance. The jigsaw model for midwifery care is introduced and explained, providing a framework to explore each aspect of antenatal care described in subsequent chapters. Chapter 2 explores the options available for women. It outlines the models of care and the range of professionals who may contribute to it. Chapter 3 describes the booking history and how the midwife can involve the woman in decisions about her care. Chapters 4 and 5 explore how maternal health can be optimized and monitored throughout pregnancy, and Chapter 6 focuses specifically on women's emotional wellbeing during pregnancy. Chapters 7 and 8 examine the various blood tests that may be offered to women and how antenatal screening for fetal abnormality is approached. Chapter 9 explores how the wellbeing of the growing fetus is monitored during pregnancy. This volume concludes with Chapter 10, which discusses how women can prepare for the birth and how the midwife facilitates this process. This book therefore prepares the reader to provide safe, evidence-based, woman-centred maternity care. Subsequent books in the series explore contemporary intrapartum and postnatal care for women and their families, exploring the role of the midwife as a member of the multi-professional team.

National Maternity Review (2016) Better Births. Improving outcomes of maternity services in England. Available at: https://www.england.nhs.uk/wp-content/uploads/2016/02/national-maternity-review-report.pdf

Sheffield and Bournemouth 2017

Helen Baston
Jenny Hall

Acknowledgements

In the process of writing, there are always people behind the scenes who support or add to the development of the book. We would specifically like to thank Mary Seager, formerly Senior Commissioning Editor at Elsevier, for her initial vision, support and prompting to turn the journal articles from *The Practising Midwife* into a readable volume. This project has now further developed with the insight and patience of Veronika Watkins and Alison Taylor. In addition, neither of us could have completed this second edition without the love, support and endless patience of our amazing families. To you, we owe our greatest gratitude.

Introduction

Introduction

This book is the second in the *Midwifery Essentials* series aimed at student midwives and those who support them in clinical practice. It focuses on antenatal care for low-risk women beginning with how antenatal care is organized and then taking the reader through the pregnancy journey. Scenarios are used throughout the book to facilitate learning and assist the reader to apply this knowledge to their own practice areas. In particular, one woman, Joanna, is followed throughout the course of her pregnancy to illustrate how different issues become more pertinent or prominent at different times along the way. The focus for contemporary maternity care is choice and continuity of care within a safe and personalized service (National Maternity Review 2016). The focus of this book is to explore ways in which this aspiration can become a reality for women and their families.

The aim of this introductory chapter is:

- To introduce the 'jigsaw model' for exploring effective midwifery practice.

The jigsaw model (Fig. 1.1) is used throughout the book, except for Chapter 2, which provides a general introduction to the various models of antenatal care currently available.

Midwifery care model

One of the purposes of this series is to consider the care of women and their babies from an holistic viewpoint. This means considering the care from a physical, emotional, psychological, spiritual, social and cultural context. To do this we have devised a jigsaw model of care that will encourage the reader to consider individual aspects of care, while recognizing that these aspects go to make up part of the whole person being cared for.

This model will be used to reflect on the clinical scenarios described in the chapters. It shows the dimensions for effective maternity care, and each should be considered during the assessment, planning, implementation and evaluation of an aspect of care.

The pieces of the jigsaw (Fig. 1.1) clearly interlink with each other, and each is needed for the provision of safe, holistic care. When one is missing,

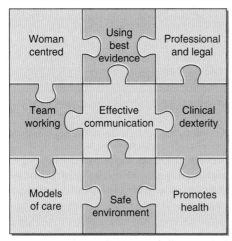

Fig. 1.1 Jigsaw model: dimensions of effective midwifery care.

the picture will be incomplete and care will not reach its potential. Each aspect of the model is described next in more detail. It is recommended that when an aspect of midwifery care is being evaluated, each piece of the jigsaw is addressed. Consider the questions pertaining to each piece of the jigsaw, and work through those that are relevant to the clinical situation you face.

Woman-centred care

The provision of woman-centred care was one of the central messages of the policy document *Changing Childbirth* (Department of Health 1993) which turned the focus of maternity care from meeting the needs of the professionals to listening and responding to the aspirations of women. This is further enforced in the *National Service Framework* (Department of Health 2004) and *Maternity Matters* (Department of Health 2007) and reflected in *Better Births* (National Maternity Review 2016). The provision of woman-centred care is also reflected in an expectation of the National Institute for Health and Care Excellence (NICE 2008, 2017) and is an expectation of midwifery practice and pre-registration education (NMC 2009). When considering particular aspects of care, the questions that need to be addressed to ensure that the woman's care is woman-centred include:

+ Was the woman involved in the development of her care plan and its subsequent implementation?

+ Should her family or carers also be involved?
+ How can I ensure that she remains involved in further decisions about her care?
+ What are the implications of undertaking or not undertaking this procedure on this particular woman or baby?
+ Are there any factors that I need to consider that might influence the results of this procedure for this woman and their impact on her?
+ How does this procedure fit in with the woman's hopes, expectations and meanings?
+ Is now the most appropriate time to undertake this procedure?

Using best evidence

A growing body of research evidence is available to inform the postnatal care we provide. We have a duty to apply this knowledge, as the NMC Code states: 'always practice in line with the best available evidence' (NMC 2015:7). The use of evidence in practise is complex and multi-faceted, and its application is influenced by many factors, including its authority and consensus amongst colleagues (Kennedy et al 2012).

Questions that need to be addressed when exploring the evidence base of care include:

+ What is already known about this aspect of care?
+ What is the justification for the choices made about care?
+ What is the research evidence available on this procedure/test?
+ Do local guidelines reflect best evidence?
+ Was a midwife involved in development of local/national guidelines?
+ Who represents users of maternity services on groups where guidelines are developed?
+ What midwifery research project has your trust been involved in?
+ Where do you go first to identify sources of best evidence?

Professional and legal

Women need to feel confident that the midwives who care for them are working within a framework that supports safe practice. Midwives who practise in the United Kingdom must adhere to the guidance of the NMC. The Code (NMC 2015:02) states:

> UK nurses and midwives must act in line with the Code, whether they are providing direct care to individuals, groups or communities or bringing their professional knowledge to bear on nursing and midwifery practice in other roles, such as leadership, education or research [...] This commitment to professional standards is fundamental to being part of a profession.

Midwives are therefore required to comply with English law and the rules and regulations of their employers.

Questions that need to be addressed to ensure that the woman's care fulfils statutory obligations include:

- Is this procedure expected to be an integral part of education before qualification?
- How do the midwives rules relate to this care/test?
- Which NMC proficiencies relate to this care/test?
- How does the NMC Code relate to this care/test?
- Is there any other NMC guidance applicable to this care/test?
- Are there any national or international guidelines for this care/test?
- Are there any legal issues underpinning the use of this care/test?

Team working

Although midwives are the experts in low-risk antenatal care, they remain reliant on a number of other workers to provide a comprehensive, safe service. Midwives work as part of a team of professionals who each bring particular skills and perspectives to the care of women and their families. The NMC Code requires registrants to 'support students' and colleagues' learning to help them develop their professional competence and confidence' (2015:09). It also states:

- Respect the skills, expertise and contributions of your colleagues, referring matters to them when appropriate.
- Maintain effective communication with colleagues.
- Keep colleagues informed when you are sharing the care of individuals with other healthcare professionals and staff.
- Work with colleagues to evaluate the quality of your work and that of the team.
- Work with colleagues to preserve the safety of those receiving care.
- Share information to identify and reduce risk.
- Be supportive of colleagues who are encountering health or performance problems. However, this support must never compromise or be at the expense of patient or public safety (NMC 2015:08).

Questions that need to be addressed to ensure that the woman's care makes appropriate use of the multi-professional team include:

- Does this test fall within my role?
- Have I acknowledged the limitations of my professional knowledge?
- Who else will need to be involved to interpret the results?
- Where should these results be recorded for all to see?
- Who will I involve if the results are outside normal parameters?
- How can I facilitate effective team working for this woman?

+ Will another person be required to assist with this care?
+ When will this person be available, and how can I access them?

Effective communication

Central to any interaction between a woman and the midwife is effective communication. It is essential that the midwife is aware of the cues she is giving to the woman during the care she provides. Time is often pressured in midwifery, both in the community and hospital setting, but it is important to convey to the woman that she is the focus of your attention. Taking time to explain what you are going to do, and why, is crucial if she is going to trust that you are acting in her best interest. Questions that need to be addressed to ensure that effective communication is achieved before, during and after any aspect of antenatal care include:

+ What information needs to be given in order for the woman to choose whether this is the right decision for her?
+ Has she given consent?
+ Is she clear what the care/test entails?
+ In what ways could the information be given?
+ What should be said during the care/test?
+ What should be observed in the woman's behaviour during the care/test?
+ What should be communicated to the woman after the care/test?
+ How and where should recording of the care/test and its results be made?

Clinical dexterity

Midwifery is a profession that requires the practitioner to have a range of knowledge and a repertoire of clinical skills. The midwife continues to learn new skills throughout her working life and is accountable for maintaining and developing her practice as new ways of working are introduced, 'keep your knowledge and skills up to date, taking part in appropriate and regular learning and professional development activities that aim to maintain and develop your competence and improve your performance' (NMC 2015:17).

Questions that need to be addressed to ensure that the woman's care is provided with clinical dexterity include:

+ How has practice changed since I started my education programme/ qualified as a midwife?
+ Can I practise this skill in other ways?
+ How has my previous experience influenced how I approach this procedure today?
+ How can I be sure I am carrying this out correctly?

+ Are there opportunities for practising this skill elsewhere?
+ Who can I observe to explore alternative ways of doing this?

Models of care

A midwife works in many settings and in a range of maternity care systems. For example, she may work independently providing holistic client-centred care, or she may work within a large tertiary centre providing care for women with specific health needs. The models of care can be influential in determining the care that a woman may receive, who from and when. Midwives need to consider the most appropriate ways that care can be delivered so that they can influence future development in the best interests of women and their families.

Questions that need to be addressed to ensure that the impact of the way that care is provided is acknowledged include:

+ How long has care been provided in this way?
+ How is the maternity service organized?
+ Which professional groups are involved in the provision of this service?
+ How is this procedure/care influenced by the model of care provided?
+ How does this model of care impact on the carers?
+ How does this model of care impact on the woman and her family?
+ Is this the best way to provide care from a professional point of view?

Safe environment

Midwives providing antenatal care need to ensure that the environment in which they work supports safe and effective working practices and protects the woman and her family from harm. The NMC Code states that 'you must maintain the knowledge and skills for safe and effective practice' (NMC 2015:07). The midwife must ensure that the care she gives does not compromise the safety of women and their families. She must therefore create and maintain a safe working environment at all times, whether in a woman's home, a midwifery-led unit or a tertiary maternity service.

Questions that need to be addressed to ensure that the woman's care is provided in a safe environment include:

+ Can the woman be assured that her confidentiality will be maintained?
+ Does the woman understand the implications of giving her consent to this procedure?
+ Are there facilities to ensure that her privacy and dignity are maintained?
+ Is there somewhere to wash hands?
+ Is there an appropriate place to dispose of waste?

- Is the equipment appropriately maintained and free from contamination?
- Is the space adequate to allow ease of movement around the woman without invading her personal space?
- What risks are involved in this procedure/care and how have they been addressed?
- Are there any risks to the person undertaking this procedure/care?
- Is this environment safe for others who might come into the room?

Promotes health

Providing care for women and their families presents a unique opportunity to influence the health and wellbeing of the public. Midwives must capitalize on their contacts with women to help them achieve a healthy pregnancy and birth and promote lifestyle choices that will benefit women, babies and families in the future.

Questions that need to be addressed to ensure that the woman's care promotes health include:

- Is this procedure/care going to help her or harm her or her baby in any way?
- What are the opportunities to use this procedure to educate her/her family on healthy behaviours?
- What resources can women and families access to help them make healthy lifestyle choices?
- Has enough time been allocated to this aspect of care to make the most of the opportunities to promote healthy living?
- Who else should I involve to ensure that the woman and her family get the best possible advice in this situation?

The book begins with a chapter focusing on the models of antenatal care. The models of care available and accessed by women can have a significant influence on her experience of pregnancy. The following chapters then use the jigsaw model to explore scenarios from practice. Thus the reader is provided with a structure with which to reflect on her care and that of the multi-professional team in which she works. Each chapter includes a range of activities designed to enable the midwife to contextualize the information within her own practice, applying her continually developing knowledge to her own circumstances. The chapters are written so that they can be accessed without having read the previous ones, although we hope you will find the whole book relevant and thought provoking. Enjoy!

References

Department of Health, 1993. Changing childbirth: Report of the Expert Maternity Group Pt. II; Report of the Expert Maternity Group Pt.1. London, Department of Health.

Department of Health, 2004. National Service Framework for children, young people and maternity services. Standard 11. Maternity Services, London, Department of Health.

Department of Health, 2007. Maternity matters: choice, access and continuity of care in a safe service. London, Department of Health.

Kennedy, H., Doig, E., Hackley, B., et al., 2012. The midwifery two-step: a study on evidence-based midwifery practice. J. Midwifery Womens Health 57 (5), 454–460.

National Institute for Health and Care Excellence NICE, 2008, updated 2017. Antenatal care: for uncomplicated pregnancies. CG62. https://www.nice.org.uk/guidance/cg62. (Accessed 28 October 2017).

National Maternity Review, 2016. Better Births. Improving outcomes of maternity services in England. Available at: https://www.england.nhs.uk/wp-content/uploads/2016/02/national-maternity-review-report.pdf. (Accessed 3 October 2016).

Nursing and Midwifery Council, 2009. Standards for pre-registration midwifery education. https://www.nmc.org.uk/standards/additional-standards/standards-for-pre-registration-midwifery-education/.

Nursing and Midwifery Council, 2015. The code: professional standards of practice and behaviour for nurses and midwives. https://www.nmc.org.uk/globalassets/sitedocuments/nmc-publications/nmc-code.pdf.

Models of antenatal care: the options available

TRIGGER SCENARIO

Joanna is 28 years old and lives with her partner, Louis, in a second-floor flat in the outskirts of a major city. She works full time and enjoys reading and cooking in her spare time. Joanna is in good health and was surprised when her usually regular menstrual cycle was interrupted. A pregnancy test bought from the local supermarket confirmed that she was pregnant, and she thought long and hard about finding the right way to break the news to Louis. He was shocked, but delighted and this unplanned but very much wanted pregnancy began its 9-month course.

Models of care

Although it is possible to describe various models of antenatal care, in reality, each individual system of healthcare provision will inevitably be a variation on a theme. Within each locality there may be a range of options available to a woman and these may also vary depending on where she lives or on the level of perceived risk her pregnancy presents. The recent review of maternity services in England, *Better Births* (National Maternity Review 2016), and that in Scotland, *The Best Start* (Scottish Gov 2017), highlight that the expected approach should be individualized to the woman. National Institute for Health and Care Excellence (NICE) (2008, 2017) guidelines state that continuity of care should be provided by a small group of healthcare professionals. In principle, there should be equal opportunity for models of care; however, in reality, not all options are available everywhere. Hence the following descriptions provide a broad outline of the main models of care in the United Kingdom, which are mirrored in many other countries, rather than an exhaustive list of every permutation available.

Principles of antenatal care

Women need to receive realistic information about the care they will receive and what the limits of reproductive technologies are. Central to women's expectations is some continuity with the care provider, combined with effective communication and the provision of information (Galle et al 2015).

The following list provides an overview of what antenatal care aims to achieve:

+ Diagnose pregnancy
+ Facilitate the development of a relationship with the woman and her carer that enables effective communication
+ Evaluation of the woman's previous and current obstetric, medical and social history to establish appropriate care patterns for the wellbeing of herself and the unborn baby
+ Provide evidence-based information about choices for care in a way that is meaningful to the woman and her partner
+ Confirm and monitor maternal and fetal wellbeing throughout pregnancy, referring to appropriate specialist help if not within normal ranges
+ Prepare the woman and her birthing partner for labour and parenthood
+ Provide an accessible source of support to pregnant women

A number of objectives are required to meet each of these aims. Many will be generic, but some will be specific to the individual needs of each family unit. The content and provision of antenatal care will be discussed in subsequent chapters in this book.

Access to antenatal care

Most women access maternity services via their general practitioner (GP), although the proportion of women who see the midwife first has increased and was 29% in 2014 compared with 20% in 2010 (Redshaw & Henderson 2015). It is unlikely now for a family doctor to continue to undertake antenatal care for a woman with a straightforward pregnancy. They will, however, work closely with midwives as needed, as family doctors remain uniquely placed to offer care for women and their families over a number of years rather than just a few months (Sikorski et al 1995). Women can access midwives as the first point of contact when they find out they are pregnant, and this is policy recommendation in Scotland (National Health Service (NHS) Quality Improvement Scotland 2009).

NICE (2008, 2017) recommends that women should have a booking appointment by 10 weeks of pregnancy; 91% of women who responded to the National Maternity Survey had booked by 12 weeks (Redshaw & Henderson 2015). This first appointment comprises a detailed assessment of previous medical and obstetric history, during which the midwife identifies any potential risks that necessitate referring the woman to a specialist clinic at the hospital.

Schedules of antenatal care over time

> **Activity**
>
> Access your copy of the standards for competence for registered midwives (Nursing and Midwifery Council (NMC) 2017a). Read them and identify which apply to your role within antenatal care.

To appreciate the range of antenatal care provision today, it is useful to see it in the context of how care has been organized historically.

The pattern of antenatal care in the United Kingdom was originally laid down in a report from the Ministry of Health in 1929. It stated that women should be seen every fortnight from 28 weeks of pregnancy and then weekly from 36 weeks until the baby is born. However, this regimented pattern of care was challenged by Hall et al (1980) who concluded that the detection of asymptotic problems during routine antenatal care was low and that the number of visits for women with a low risk of complications could be considerably reduced. Later, a randomized controlled trial was conducted that compared traditional care (13 visits) with 'new style' care (7 visits) (Sikorski et al 1996). The results demonstrated that in reality there was less difference between the mean number of visits that women actually received than anticipated (10.8 visits compared with 8.6 in the study group). They evaluated both clinical outcomes and client satisfaction. No statistical significance was found between clinical outcomes, but women were more dissatisfied if they had fewer visits, as they valued regular contact with professionals.

Midwives also had some reservations about reduced schedules of care, in particular, regarding the detection of raised blood pressure and developing a relationship with the woman (Sanders et al 1999). In a Swedish study (Hildingsson et al 2002), women preferred more antenatal visits if it was their first pregnancy or if they had a previous negative reproductive experience. Older women and those with more than two children preferred fewer visits. The World Health Organization (WHO) has taken a proactive stance regarding the scheduling of antenatal care. In a multi-centre trial involving 24,678 women, a model comprising a screening checklist and a basic package of four antenatal visits was implemented and evaluated (Villar et al 2001). The content of each visit was also specified, and outcomes revealed minimal differences between the study and control groups for maternal, fetal and neonatal outcomes (Villar & Bergsjo 2002). The conclusions of this trial are supported by a comparative systematic review of alternative models of antenatal care for low-risk pregnancies (Dowswell et al 2015), which again highlighted that maternal satisfaction is often diminished when contact with health professionals is reduced.

Schedules of antenatal care vary between individual trusts, midwives, obstetricians and women. Although a general ideal pattern may be part of written guidance for practice, it is appropriate that care reflects the individual needs of women. National guidance recommends 7 antenatal appointments for multiparous women and 10 for primiparous women (NICE 2008, 2017).

Who provides antenatal care?

In a national survey (Redshaw & Henderson 2015), 58% were cared for exclusively by midwives in the antenatal period, compared with 49% of women in 2007. Doctors at the maternity unit were involved in the care of 31% of women, and 15% of women had at least one appointment with a GP. Around 98% of women receive some midwifery care in the antenatal period, and 36% have had continuity with the same person (Care Quality Commission 2015).

Although globally midwives are able to provide total care to childbearing women, their sphere of practice is normal childbirth, and in the UK they are bound by the law and standards (NMC 2017a) to refer women to an appropriate health professional if their condition deviates from normal parameters. Women will continue to require midwifery care in such circumstances, and it is the cooperation and respect between members of a multidisciplinary team that will enhance the woman's experience of her care.

Midwives

Activity

Access the document: Opportunities for Africa's newborns (The Patnership for Maternal, Newborn and Child Health 2006): http://www.who.int/pmnch/media/publications/oanfullreport.pdf.

Look at the box, 'The essential elements of a focused approach to antenatal care' on page 53.

Are these relevant to your own area of practice? How would they help you provide women-centred care?

Midwives are the experts in the provision of antenatal care for women at low risk of complications. The international definition of a midwife is agreed to be:

> The midwife is recognised as a responsible and accountable professional who works in partnership with women to give the necessary support, care and advice during pregnancy, labour and the postpartum period, to conduct births on the midwife's own responsibility and to provide care for the newborn and the infant.

(International Confederation of Midwives (ICM) 2017)

In recent years it has been acknowledged that midwives and midwifery care has a positive impact on women's and babies' wellbeing (Renfrew et al 2014), and there is an aim to increase the numbers of midwives globally. Midwifery care can be provided in partnership with either a family doctor or an obstetrician, or as part of a multi-disciplinary team, which could include a health visitor, community psychiatric nurse or social services teams. It has been highlighted that globally 'every woman needs a midwife and some need a doctor too' (Sandall 2012). The role of the midwife as the lead professional for women with uncomplicated pregnancies is recognized (National Maternity Review 2016; NICE 2008, 2017; Scottish Gov 2017), if not universally adopted.

> **Activity**
> Access the rest of the definition of a midwife from the ICM website. Consider how the definition is applicable to you and your practice.

Community-based midwives generally provide the majority of antenatal care to women with uncomplicated pregnancies. This care usually takes place in community health centres or GPs' surgeries and sometimes in shopping centres or the woman's family home. Within most maternity systems there are midwives who work mostly in the community, birth centre or hospital settings, although some work across all areas. Some midwives work independently from the NHS and are employed by women for a fee, usually fixed. Women who are able to access the services of an independent midwife can then usually expect continuity of care from a known carer.

Hospital midwives provide care for women attending antenatal clinics for specialist tests and investigations or for monitoring of more complicated pregnancies. Clinics, where consultants from a range of specialties attend, provide care for pregnant women who also have underlying medical problems. Some hospitals have antenatal day care units where women can attend for assessment and care without having to stay in hospital overnight. A minority of women will need to stay in hospital at some point during their pregnancy, and midwives work with obstetricians and other healthcare professionals to plan care that meets their unique needs.

Consultant obstetricians

Although many women may have a named consultant for their obstetric care, it is unlikely that they will receive much direct care from them, unless there are complicated aspects to the pregnancy. Consultant obstetricians usually have a team of doctors working with them at varying levels of obstetric training who assist with the support of women during the antenatal period. Some consultants also work in private practice. Midwives should be able to refer directly to obstetricians as required if a problem arises in an otherwise previously normal pregnancy.

Specialists

As technology advances, more women are becoming pregnant who would previously have remained childless. Conditions such as cystic fibrosis, cancer, diabetes and cardiac anomalies now complicate pregnancies that hitherto would not have been conceived. Advances in genetic technology in relation to pregnancy have also influenced antenatal care for those who have a complex family history. The care of such women needs to be closely coordinated and monitored and will require a plan of action that involves senior professionals, including, for example, paediatricians, anaesthetists and intensive therapy staff. Care is often provided in joint clinics where specialists and obstetricians can work together with the woman and midwives to provide coordinated care that will meet her individual needs.

Support workers

The title and responsibilities of a midwife are protected by law in the UK (NMC 2017b). This means that midwives cannot delegate their role to anyone other than a registered medical practitioner. However, there are aspects of the midwives' role that can be supported by appropriately trained healthcare support workers ranging from clerical and housekeeping duties to direct client contact in the promotion of public health (Sandall & Mansfield 2007). Maternity support workers should work within clearly defined protocols and the Royal College of Midwives' guide that maternity support workers:

> …*do not assess mothers and babies or make clinical judgements or decisions or initiate interventions.*
>
> (Royal College of Midwives (RCM) 2016:5)

In Scotland there are competencies for maternity support carers in the health service, but this is yet to be agreed across the NHS in England.

Health visitors

The role of the health visitor is a specialist nurse who focuses on the care of families with children under 5 years of age. Although not directly responsible for antenatal care, it is part of their remit to introduce themselves to pregnant women in the antenatal period. They may already be involved in monitoring the health and wellbeing of the unborn baby's siblings. It is suggested that this early contact may have an impact on reducing inequality of health in the future (Christie 2016). In some areas, health visitors also take on specialist roles, for example, supporting teenage parents, and they often contribute to preparation for parenthood classes. Midwives in the community will work closely with the health visitor to provide support to vulnerable women in their locality.

Social services

Some women will benefit from the additional services provided by social workers or family liaison workers, particularly those women whose social circumstances are complicated by poverty, abuse and disadvantage. Such vulnerable women may include teenage parents, homeless women, refugees or asylum seekers, victims of domestic abuse and victims of substance misuse. It is particularly important that their care is carefully coordinated and that they have a named midwife who has an in-depth insight into their unique history and personal challenges. *Better Births* (National Maternity Review 2016) states that community hubs should be established where maternity care takes place alongside those family support and social support service providers.

Activity

Find out your main contacts for vulnerable women in your locality and how you would make contact with them.

Other professionals

Some women with a particular disability or health need would benefit from the contribution of an occupational therapist or physiotherapist during the antenatal period to continue activities of daily living. Women also need to get ready for life with a new baby, and these practitioners may be involved in the antenatal period to support in these preparations. For women with known psychiatric conditions, a community-based psychiatric nurse may be involved in care during the antenatal period and continue this care after the birth of the baby. In addition, specialist consultant midwives may provide expert support and advice for some women with complicated circumstances, for example, fear of childbirth.

In all these cases the community midwife will usually be the lead practitioner for care for the woman and will liaise with the other professionals on how to best meet her needs and those of her baby. It is beneficial to find out how to refer women in these circumstances in each locality, as provision of care may be through different service providers.

Activity

Next time you care for a woman in late pregnancy, consult her notes and identify how many professionals she has seen during her pregnancy.

What do you think is the minimum number of professionals a woman would need to see during the antenatal period? How would this link with the principles of holistic, individualized and continuous care?

Models of care

A range of healthcare professionals contribute to the provision of maternity services. Combined with a variety of models of care, the organization of maternity care is unique to each locality. A plethora of different schemes have been designed to meet the recommendations of various government policies and reports such as *Changing Childbirth* (Department of Health (DH) 1993), *Maternity Matters* (DH 2007) and, now, *Better Births* (National Maternity Review 2016) and *The Best Start* in Scotland (Scottish Gov 2017). These have all aimed to provide more continuity of care, individualized care, more community-based services and better use of the midwives' skills. An audit of organization of current services in England pointed to only 15% of trust boards where women are provided schemes of continuity of caregiver (National Maternity and Perinatal Audit (NMPA) Project Team 2017). These schemes have often been implemented and evaluated alongside the 'traditional' system. With the availability of so many models of care, it is important that all new services are carefully evaluated to monitor not only the impact on women but also on those providing the service; being able to cultivate relationships with women and colleagues and a passion for midwifery 'transcends models of care' (Crowther et al 2016:47).

Midwife-led care

Where women have straightforward pregnancies, in this model of care, midwives are the lead professional. Women who are cared for within this scheme need never see a medical practitioner unless the progress of pregnancy deviates from normal. Criteria for being and remaining at low risk of complications, such as those of NICE (2008, 2017), are employed to ensure that there are clear pathways of referral should a woman need to have additional specialist maternity care. Care is usually based entirely in the community, although some midwife-led units are attached to larger obstetric maternity units that provide antenatal and postnatal care as well as intrapartum care. Community-based midwives work almost exclusively in the primary care setting providing antenatal and postnatal care, with a rota for 24-hour on-call support for home births.

Continuity-of-care models

There have been many different ways in which maternity services organize and deliver a midwifery-led approach to care (e.g. Sandall et al 2016; Wraight et al 1993). The main focus of team-based midwifery when first introduced was to provide continuity of care from a known carer; hence teams of midwives were created to cover antenatal, intrapartum and postnatal care for a caseload of women. Such teams usually comprised a defined group of midwives who worked from the community, in private practice or from an NHS hospital trust. One of the first examples of team midwifery was the 'Know your midwife' scheme which operated in Tooting between 1983 and 1985. Low-risk women were randomized to receive most of their care from either one of a team of four midwives or conventional hospital care (Flint & Poulengeris 1987). The scheme was associated with increased satisfaction with antenatal care and feeling more prepared for parenthood. Thirty years later, initiatives continue to be launched with the aim of providing care throughout the childbirth continuum by known caregivers, as recommended by *Better Births* (National Maternity Review 2016). Continuity of care is associated with reduced intervention (Sandall et al 2013) and enhanced safety (National Maternity Review 2016), but may be difficult to facilitate where staff work long shifts or part-time hours. In some areas, a group of midwives may link with a particular consultant or a geographical location.

Activity

Access https://www.england.nhs.uk/wp-content/uploads/2017/03/nhs-guidance-maternity-services-v1.pdf and consider how the maternity service where you work meets the requirements of continuity of carer outlined on page 36.

Group practice

An example of this innovative model of care is the Albany Midwifery Practice (NHS England 2016; Reid 2002). It was an independently run, self-managed group of seven midwives and a practice manager contracted into the NHS (hence women did not have to pay for the service). Continuity of carer was offered by two known midwives throughout the childbirth continuum, although the midwives did not work in fixed pairs. This practice is no longer running, but such models are recommended to be the way forward for maternity care (NHS England 2016). A significant difference between the team and group practice model is that midwives in the latter are only on call for women in their own caseload.

Caseload midwifery

Partnership caseload practice schemes have evolved considerably over time. There has been the BUMPS (Birth Under Midwifery Practice Scheme) described and evaluated by Benjamin et al (2001) which consisted of three pairs of midwives. They provided total care to a caseload of women attached to a family doctor practice, with each midwife supporting in labour approximately 40 women per year. Antenatally, women were cared for by the same two midwives throughout their pregnancy. Compared with the traditional model of care, women cared for under BUMPS had more home births, fewer epidurals, more normal births and less induction of labour. They were more likely to go hospital early and be cared for by a midwife they knew. The practice no longer continues, but various similar models have evolved globally.

Independent midwifery practice

Midwives may practice in a range of settings (ICM 2017), having completed a programme of preparation and gained the requisite qualifications. Some midwives choose to work independently from the NHS and offer a flexible, personalized service to women in their own homes. Sometimes independent midwives work with another midwife for mutual support and on-call cover. Women can contract for all or part of their care depending on their requirements. However, independent midwifery in the UK has been threatened as professional indemnity insurance (PII) is now a pre-requisite of professional registration (NMC 2015). Independent midwives have previously got around their inability to hold insurance by informing women when they contract to care for them that they do not have PII and what the implication of this might mean. Some midwives still practice independently just for antenatal and postnatal care, whereas others have joined into small businesses and are contracted into the NHS and thus covered through NHS indemnity schemes. The situation remains complex, and it is now more difficult to provide care in this way. All midwives, wherever they practice in the UK, must adhere to the NMC standards (NMC 2017a) and the Code for Nurses and Midwives (NMC 2015) and have adequate PII.

Activity

Joanna's last menstrual period (LMP) was 15/8/17. What is her expected date of delivery (EDD)? Find out what models of antenatal care are available in your locality.

Shared care

A traditional model of antenatal care is when care is shared between the hospital obstetrician (and potentially other medical specialists) and the family doctor and midwife in primary care. Women may attend the hospital for specialist clinics but still have the majority of their care in the community until the birth is either approaching or post-term, when their pregnancy may be reviewed by a member of the obstetric team at the hospital.

Integrated care

Some obstetric units employ midwives to work in both hospital and community settings within the same working week. This integrated model requires the midwife to be up to date with the full repertoire of midwifery skills, as she may be supporting a woman undergoing induction of labour for pre-eclampsia one day and the next be helping another woman express breast milk at home. Midwives have always been required to be able to practice the whole range of their remit, especially in an emergency. For example, a woman attending antenatal clinic in the community may unexpectedly go into premature labour, and the attending community midwife will need to provide competent care and support. This way of working ensures that the maternity unit has a flexible workforce able to meet the unpredictable workload demands of the service. This is particularly important in small units where there may not be a large workforce to rely on if there is a sudden influx of demand or a shortfall of staff. It can be very rewarding for midwives to work in this way, but it can also be exhausting to work a mixture of different day and night duties in the same week.

Consultant care

Some women with complex pregnancies will need to have their antenatal progress closely supervised by a consultant obstetrician and other senior colleagues. This care will take place at the hospital where facilities are available for detailed monitoring.

Activity

Consider each model of care. What are the implications, the advantages and disadvantages of each model for:
- Women and families
- Midwives
- Other health professionals
- The trust organization
- Student midwives

However, the woman should still be given the opportunity to develop a relationship with her community midwife who will also support her in the postnatal period.

Group antenatal care

In some maternity services group antenatal care has been introduced, whereby a group of pregnant women meet regularly (about 8 to 10 times over the pregnancy for up to 2 hours at a time) and midwives facilitate their care in the group setting. A meta-analysis of the evidence demonstrated little difference in outcomes between the usual individual pattern of care and group antenatal methods (Catling et al 2015). However, this highlighted that there are few studies and further robust evidence is required before such models can be described as effective and satisfactory for women.

One study in Australia identified that when group antenatal care was introduced within a case-loading practice, this interfered with the development of relationships between midwives and the women (Allen et al 2015). However, in a randomized study in the United States, group care was demonstrated to have a positive impact, reducing the incidence of preterm births. In addition, women's knowledge and satisfaction increased and higher breastfeeding rates were seen (Ickovics et al 2007).

Another investigation group combined physical care and education and concluded that the format met both physical and clinical requirements and prepared the parents for birth, but not for parenting (Andersson et al 2012). It is evident that further work is required to establish if there are benefits of group care over individual care and how they relate to parental satisfaction. Current UK guidance mandates that the environment of antenatal care should be one where women are able 'to discuss sensitive issues such as domestic violence, sexual abuse, psychiatric illness and recreational drug use' (NICE 2008, 2017); therefore whichever model of care is provided, opportunity for privacy should be available.

Activity

Consider what the effect of group antenatal care may be on disclosure of previous abortion, mental health concerns, sexual abuse or domestic abuse.

Find out more about asking questions about these challenging circumstances.

REFLECTION ON THE TRIGGER SCENARIO

Look back on the trigger scenario.

> Joanna is 28 years old and lives with her partner, Louis, in a second-floor flat in the outskirts of a major city. She works full time and enjoys reading and cooking in her spare time. Joanna is in good health and was surprised when her usually regular menstrual cycle was interrupted. A pregnancy test bought from the local supermarket confirmed that she was pregnant, and she thought long and hard about finding the right way to break the news to Louis. He was shocked, but delighted and this unplanned but very much wanted pregnancy began its 9-month course.

Practice point

Joanna is pregnant for the first time and appears to be in good health. She therefore should be able to choose to have care that meets her needs. It is important that women are given appropriate information so that they may consider which type of care they want to access. For example, midwives are the experts in normal pregnancy and birth, and therefore if a woman does not have any known risk factors, she should be able to access midwife-led care. Timely access to the most appropriate type of care is particularly important where a pregnancy is unplanned, as there may be delay in seeking professional support.

Further questions specific to this scenario include:

1. How can Joanna find information about who to go to now that she knows she is pregnant?
2. What information do shop-bought pregnancy tests include about accessing maternity services?
3. What proportion of pregnancies are unplanned?
4. What provision is there where you work for choice of care provider?
5. Can women at low risk of complications go through their entire pregnancy and birth without seeing a medical practitioner?

Conclusion

Joanna has faced the hurdle of telling her partner that they are going to have a baby. She is probably unaware of the many systems and professionals that exist to support her throughout pregnancy. It is important for her to be provided this information so that she may choose the most appropriate model to meet her needs. Midwives work in a range of settings with professionals whose roles and skills are complementary. Effective team working and mutual respect will enhance the woman's experience of her care.

References

Allen, J., Kildea, S., Stapleton, H., et al., 2015. How does group antenatal care function within a caseload midwifery model? A critical ethnographic analysis. Midwifery 31 (5), 489–497.

Andersson, E., Christensson, K., Hildingsson, I., 2012. Parents' experiences and perceptions of group-based antenatal care in four clinics in Sweden. Midwifery 28 (4), 442–448.

Benjamin, Y., Walsh, D., Taub, N., 2001. A comparison of partnership caseload midwifery care with conventional team midwifery care: labour and birth outcomes. Midwifery 17 (3), 234–240.

Care Quality Commission, 2015. 2015 survey of women's experiences of maternity care. Available from: http://www.cqc.org.uk/sites/default/files/20151215b_mat15_statistical_release.pdf.

Catling, C.J., Medley, N., Foureur, M., et al., 2015. Group versus conventional antenatal care for women. Cochrane Database Syst. Rev. (2), Art. No.: CD007622, doi:10.1002/14651858.CD007622.pub3.

Christie, L., 2016. The importance of the antenatal home visit by the health visitor. J. of Health Visiting 4 (3), 142–148.

Crowther, S., Hunter, B., Mcara-Couper, J., et al., 2016. Sustainability and resilience in midwifery: a discussion paper. Midwifery 40, 40–48.

Department of Health, 1993. Changing Childbirth Part 1: Report of the Expert Maternity Group. London, HMSO.

Department of Health, 2007. Maternity Matters: Choice, Access and Continuity of Care in a Safe Service. London, DH.

Dowswell, T., Carroli, G., Duley, L., et al., 2015. Alternative versus standard packages of antenatal care for low-risk pregnancy. Cochrane Database Syst. Rev. (7), Art. No.: CD000934, doi:10.1002/14651858.CD000934.pub3.

Flint, C., Poulengeris, P., 1987. The know your midwife report. South West Thames Regional Health Authority and the Wellington Foundation.

Galle, A., Van Parys, A.S., Roelens, K., et al., 2015. Expectations and satisfaction with antenatal care among pregnant women with a focus on vulnerable groups: a descriptive study in Ghent. BMC Womens Health 15, 112. doi:10.1186/s12905-015-0266-2.

Hall, M.H., Chng, P.K., Macgillivray, I., 1980. Is routine antenatal care worthwhile? Lancet 12 (7), 78–80.

Hildingsson, I., Waldenstrom, U., Radestad, I., 2002. Women's expectations on antenatal care as assessed in early pregnancy: number of visits, continuity of caregiver and general content. Acta. Obstet. Gynecol. Scand. 81 (2), 118–125.

Ickovics, J.R., Kershaw, T.S., Westdahl, C., et al., 2007. Group prenatal care and perinatal outcomes: a randomized controlled trial. Obstet. Gynecol. 110 (2 Pt 1), 330–339.

International Confederation of Midwives, 2017. International Definition of the Midwife. Available from: http://internationalmidwives.org/assets/uploads/documents/CoreDocuments/ENG%20Definition_of_the_Midwife%202017.pdf.

National Maternity Service Review, 2016. Better Births, Improving Outcomes of Maternity Services in England, A 5 Year Forward View for the Maternity Services. London, DH.

National Health Service (NHS) Quality Improvement Scotland, 2009. Pathways for maternity care. http://www.healthcareimprovementscotland.org/previous_resources/implementation_support/keeping_childbirth_natural__d.aspx.

National Institute for Health and Care Excellence (NICE), 2008, 2017. Antenatal care for uncomplicated pregnancies. clinical guideline. https://www.nice.org.uk/guidance/cg62.

NMPA Project Team, 2017. National Maternity and Perinatal Audit: organisational report 2017. RCOG London.

Nursing and Midwifery Council, 2009. Standards for pre-registration midwifery education. https://www.nmc.org.uk/standards/additional-standards/standards-for-pre-registration-midwifery-education/

Nursing and Midwifery Council, 2015. The Code for Nurses and Midwives. NMC, London.

Nursing and Midwifery Council, 2017a. Standards for competence for registered midwives. https://www.nmc.org.uk/globalassets/sitedocuments/standards/nmc-standards-for-competence-for-registered-midwives.pdf.

Nursing and Midwifery Council, 2017b. Practising as a midwife in the UK: an overview of midwifery regulation. Available from: https://www.nmc.org.uk/globalassets/sitedocuments/nmc-publications/practising-as-a-midwife-in-the-uk.pdf.

Redshaw, M., Henderson, J., 2015. Safely Delivered: A national survey of women's experience of maternity care 2014. https://www.npeu.ox.ac.uk/downloads/files/reports/Safely%20delivered%20NMS%202014.pdf.

Reid, B., 2002. The Albany midwifery practice. MIDIRS Midwifery Digest 14 (1), 118–121.

Renfrew, M., Mcfadden, A., Bastos, M., et al., 2014. Midwifery and quality care: findings from a new evidence-informed framework for maternal and newborn care. Lancet 384 (9948), 1129–1145.

Royal College of Midwives (RCM), 2016. The roles and responsibilities of MSWs. Available from: https://www.rcm.org.uk/sites/default/files/The%20Role%20and%20Responsibilities%20of%20Maternity%20Support%20Workers%20A5%2020pp_12%20Spreads_0.pdf.

Sandall, J., Jill, M., Mansfield, A., 2007. Support workers in maternity services. J. Fam. Health Care 17 (6), 191–192.

Sandall, J., 2012. Every woman needs a midwife, and some women need a doctor too. Birth 39 (4), 323–326.

Sandall, J., Soltani, H., Gates, S., et al., 2013. Midwife-led continuity models versus other models of care for childbearing women. Cochrane Database Syst. Rev. (8) Art. No.: CD004667, doi:10.1002/14651858.CD004667.pub3.

Sandall, J., Soltani, H., Gates, S., et al., 2016. Midwife-led continuity models of care compared with other models of care for women during pregnancy, birth and early parenting. Cochrane Database Syst. Rev. (4), Art. No.: CD004667, doi:10.1002/14651858.CD004667.pub5.

Sanders, J., Somerset, M., Jewell, D., et al., 1999. To see or not to see? Midwives' perceptions of reduced antenatal attendances for low-risk women. Midwifery 15 (4), 257–263.

Scottish Gov, 2017. The best start: A five-year forward plan for maternity and neonatal care in Scotland. Available from: http://www.gov.scot/Resource/0051/00513175.pdf.

Sikorski, J., Clement, S., Wilson, J., et al., 1995. A survey of health professionals' views on possible changes in the provision and organisation of antenatal care. Midwifery 11, 61–68.

Sikorski, J., Wilson, J., Clement, S., et al., 1996. A randomised controlled trial comparing two schedules of antenatal visits: the antenatal care project. Br. Med. J. 312 (7030), 546–553.

The Partnership for Maternal, Newborn and Child Health, 2006. Opportunities for Africa's newborns: Practical data, policy and programmatic support for newborn care in Africa. Available from: http://www.who.int/pmnch/media/publications/africanewborns/en/.

Villar, J., Ba'aqeel, H., Piaggio, G., et al., for the WHO Antenatal Care Trial Research Group, 2001. WHO antenatal care randomised trial for the evaluation of a new model of routine antenatal care. Lancet 357 (9268), 1551–1564.

Villar, J., Bergsjo, P., for the WHO Antenatal Care Trial Research Group, 2002. WHO Antenatal Care Randomised Control Trial: Manual for the Implementation of the New Model. World Health Organization, Geneva. WHO Opportunities for Africa's newborns. http://www.who.int/pmnch/media/publications/oanfullreport.pdf.

Wraight, A., Ball, J., Seccombe, I., Stock, J., 1993. Mapping Team Midwifery. IMS Report Series 242. Institute of Manpower Studies, Brighton.

CHAPTER 3

The booking history

TRIGGER SCENARIO

Joanna is in the first trimester of her first pregnancy. She bought a pregnancy test at home and went to see her general practitioner (GP), who gave her some general advice about what she should and should not be eating. Aware of her previous medical history, the GP told Joanna to go to the reception desk and to make an appointment for the clinic of the community midwife to undertake the 'booking'. A week later she received a package of information and a letter from the midwife confirming the appointment time and asking Joanna to produce a specimen of urine on the day of the visit.

Introduction

The initial purpose of this important first appointment with the midwife is to initiate antenatal care. Though this scenario highlights a common process of referral to midwifery services, some women may access midwives directly or have attended a pre-pregnancy clinic due to complex medical needs. However, it should be noted that when the woman confirms her pregnancy, it is also an opportunity to provide her with valuable health information, particularly about folic acid supplementation, antenatal screening, nutrition and food hygiene and lifestyle advice (National Institute for Health and Care Excellence (NICE) 2008, 2017). Early attendance will mean this advice will be provided when it is most significant. If women access midwifery services directly rather than going through a GP, this will enable them to take earlier advantage of this opportunity (Royal College of Midwives (RCM) 2011). The information and advice can be reinforced at the subsequent booking visit.

Activity

There are now numerous websites that aim to provide early pregnancy advice to women. Look at some of them and compare the information. Consider what the impact of the information could be to the women who read it and to you as a practitioner when you meet them for the first time.

Depending on the locality and model of antenatal care practised (see Chapter 1), the booking history may be conducted by the community-based midwife either in the woman's home or at the local clinic, or by a midwife at the hospital. It is usually conducted between 7 and 9 weeks of pregnancy, and NICE (2008, 2017) recommends that booking is undertaken by 10 weeks of pregnancy.

The booking visit is significant in pregnancy and is an opportunity for the woman and the midwife to get to know each other, as well as meeting the following broad aims to:

- Initiate the development of a trusting relationship between the woman and the midwife
- Commence a maternity record for the pregnancy
- Identify potential factors that may complicate the pregnancy
- Present and discuss the options for antenatal screening for the woman and fetus
- Present and discuss the options regarding the place of birth
- Undertake baseline observations and relevant blood tests
- Identify and agree on an appropriate schedule of antenatal care
- Offer lifestyle advice
- Refer to the appropriate type of pregnancy care

These will be explored broadly in turn, recognizing that locally there may be some variation. In all aspects it is to be remembered that women have the right to make the choices that are right for themselves and their babies, and information provided should be communicated in a way that will facilitate that choice (Byrom & Byrom 2017).

Developing relationships

Fundamental to all aspects of midwifery care is the need for the midwife to communicate effectively with the woman. There are aspects of the booking that the midwife can influence to help make the experience a positive one.

Place of booking

Though many women are invited to a clinic setting for a booking appointment, the place where the woman will be most comfortable and able to talk openly about how she feels is probably her own home. NICE guidance (2008, 2017) highlights the importance of accessibility of antenatal care and in an environment where women feel safe to discuss complex and sensitive concerns. There are several advantages to conducting the booking history at the woman's home address. The balance of power between the woman and health professional is more even. The woman is in her own familiar environment, on her own territory, and the midwife is a guest. Clinics and hospitals can be daunting places for women to attend. They may be associated with difficult memories and clinical smells, and there are often unfamiliar protocols to follow. Of course, many measures have been taken to make such environments friendlier and relaxed, but the privacy and familiarity associated with one's own home cannot be replicated.

It may take longer to book a woman in her own home, as such an event often involves an element of tea drinking and social chit-chat or playing with other children. Time spent by the community midwife during the booking visit getting to know the woman, not just as an individual but as a member of a family and a community, is an investment for future care. Development of trust and mutual respect at the beginning of pregnancy will enable the woman to ask questions and seek advice throughout the childbirth continuum. Worries can be discussed before they become problems. Booking a woman in her home enables the midwife to gain a deeper understanding of the woman's social circumstances, who she lives with and how supported she will be by them.

Although undertaking a booking history in the woman's home is perhaps an ideal situation, women should feel they have the choice. Some women wish to keep their pregnancy secret, for whatever reason, and would not welcome the familiar car of the midwife drawing up outside their house.

In some localities, booking takes place in a children's centre or the woman's GP surgery. Wherever the booking takes place, the midwife should have had access to the woman's medical history to ensure key issues are taken into account when subsequent care is planned.

Activity

Visit the Healthy Start website: http://www.healthystart.nhs.uk/ and identify what is available for women and who qualifies for this support. Where is the booking history undertaken in your locality? Find out if that system is universal across the region or unique to your area.

Information

The woman should be aware of what the meeting is about and what is expected of her, preferably before the meeting takes place. This should be provided at the earliest opportunity, preferably written, and include information about the number, timing and content of the appointments (NICE 2008, 2017). For example, the midwife will be asking her questions about her past medical history or asking her if there are any babies on either side of the family with congenital health problems.

If the woman is expecting to be able to provide such information, she can ask her partner if he is aware of any children on his side of the family who have a condition that might be passed on to their baby. She can ask her mother about her own health as a child and if her mother experienced any complications during her pregnancies. The community midwife or health centre may have composed a simple, friendly letter of introduction that outlines the content of the booking visit, giving her contact details if the woman needs to clarify anything or make alternative arrangements.

Communication

Midwives care for women from a range of diverse backgrounds, and it is vital that they understand each other. The Nursing and Midwifery Council (NMC) states:

> 7.2 take reasonable steps to meet people's language and communication needs…

> (NMC 2015:7)

In situations of language diversity, it is important that the booking interview is conducted with a skilled interpreter. In a review of the literature in relation to communication and cultural diversity (Robinson 2002), it is apparent that trained interpreters enhance communication, though there remains a lack of consideration around training for maternity care needs (Cambridge 2012). Many centres use telephone interpretation services. Although this method may shorten the length of the encounter, face-to-face interpretation is preferable in most cases (Locatis et al 2010).

There should be awareness, too, of any physical, sensory or learning disabilities and information provided in an appropriate form (NICE 2008, 2017). Disabled women in particular highlight the need to be listened to carefully and to be given information in a manner appropriate to their needs (Hall et al 2016).

The physical environment is also important for the process of building a relationship with the woman. Whilst in a woman's home the midwife cannot start rearranging the furniture; however, she can make best use of the layout by endeavouring to ensure that there are no physical barriers between them and that they can face each other at the same level.

We tend to get on best with people who show interest in what we are saying and who appear to be concerned about our welfare. The midwife can demonstrate that she is there to listen to the woman by sitting down with her. If she is standing up, this may convey to the woman that she is on the move and has not got time to talk. If the midwife is doing other things at the same time and not looking at the woman, this may suggest to the woman that she is not listening. This may be complicated by the positions of computers in clinic rooms, and it would be ideal to complete documentation on a laptop or tablet to be able to face the woman and have eye contact. Reflecting back what the woman has said ('so let me see if I have got this right …') before she writes it down is a useful tactic to ensure correct understanding. The woman then knows that the midwife a) had been listening and b) correctly interpreted what was said.

Clinical results should be recorded contemporaneously, but the midwife can continue to nod and smile in affirmation that she is still listening or simply say, 'Just let me write this down before I forget', to avoid appearing rude. The pressure of work can make it easy to revert to a list of closed questions, as observed in Methven's revealing study (1989). McCourt (2006) describes three styles of communication by midwives during the booking history: professional, providing expertise and guidance; disciplinary, providing expertise and surveillance; and partnership, which is much more participative and collaborative, following a conversational style rather than a ceremonial order. Eye contact is an important aspect of showing attention to another. Less eye contact is associated with inattention on the part of the listener (Rungapadiachy 1999).

It is also important to remember that some of the questions asked will be enquiring about intimate subjects, such as around periods, mental wellbeing or previous termination of pregnancies. There should be awareness that the midwife could be the first person to ask about these aspects and may raise some emotional response. It is noted that women with known mental illness do not always experience the initial encounters of the maternity service as positive, and midwives and students need to be aware of meeting these needs with appropriate referral.

Activity

Consider how you would respond should a woman not wish you to reveal any previous pregnancies to her partner or family. Are there any local policies regarding this circumstance?

Find out the referral mechanisms in your locality for women with known mental health conditions.

Completion of the maternity record

During pregnancy women are provided with maternity records that they keep and that are personal to their care. In around 60% of maternity services, a national maternity record is provided (see http://www.preg.info/PregnancyNotes/Default.aspx). They encourage the woman to contribute and be directly involved in her care. There are sections that she can complete herself and identify any questions she might have. As she holds the records throughout the pregnancy, she has the opportunity to read them in intimate detail. It is important therefore that whenever the midwife makes an entry in the records, she explains it to the woman and ensures that she knows not only what it says but also what it means. A systematic review to evaluate the effects of women carrying their own case notes during pregnancy concluded that this system improves women's feeling of control, satisfaction and the availability of antenatal records (Brown et al 2015). Further, the UK maternity policy, *Better Births* (National Maternity Review 2016) highlights the need for records to be 'interoperable' and enable the woman and her carer to communicate via a digital platform, which can also be a source of evidence-based information.

Personal information

The national maternity record begins with an important section which the woman can complete herself. It includes details about her full name and title and what she likes to be called. There are important contact details essential for the return of lost records and boxes to record the names of the professionals involved in the woman's maternity care. It also includes a place to record any communication needs and a summary box for plans for care.

Activity

What are the advantages and disadvantages of digital maternity records?

How can maternity care records be personalized for each individual woman?

In what medium is information about what to expect in pregnancy provided for women where you work?

It is on this page that the woman also records her occupation and that of the baby's father. This is important information, as occupational hazards may be associated with particular kinds of work that the midwife can give general advice about. Women may need to be encouraged to talk to their employer about reassignment of duties during their pregnancy, depending on the nature of their role. For example, if their job involves heavy lifting or standing for long periods, an alternative office role might be available during the term of the pregnancy.

Activity

Locate the Maternity Action web pages (for the UK: https://www.maternityaction.org.uk/) or your local government website to establish the rights for women around work and benefits in pregnancy.

Previous medical history

This section may also be completed by the woman. It asks the woman to indicate whether she has suffered from any of a list of illnesses. Box 3.1 provides a summary of the potential significance of each condition.

Assessment of mental wellbeing

Women with a history of mental illness have an increased risk of recurrence or fear of recurrence during pregnancy. There is also a risk of severe illness after birth, and death by suicide is a significant cause of maternal death (Knight et al 2017). The National Maternity notes include a variety of questions about previous conditions, treatments and family conditions. It also includes questions related to recent wellbeing.

Activity

Establish what questions are asked about mental wellbeing in your local antenatal documents.

Think about how you might raise these questions and consider different approaches to the same topic.

Box 3.1 Health history

- **Admission to Intensive Therapy Unit (ITU), High Dependency Unit (HDU), Accident and Emergency (A&E) recently, operations**
  Significance: To establish any recent serious medical or surgical conditions that may affect wellbeing in pregnancy. For example, cervical surgery may affect decisions regarding mode of birth; breast surgery may affect ability to breastfeed, awareness of pelvic injury is important, etc.
- **Anaesthetic problems**
  Significance: Previous failed intubation would require the presence of a consultant anaesthetist if caesarean section was needed.
- **Allergies**
  Significance: Women may have a range of allergic reactions to substances which may include latex, often used in gloves and equipment.
- **Autoimmune conditions**
  Significance: The symptoms may become better or worse during pregnancy. Will need specialist referral.
- **Back problem**
  Significance: May need assessment in relation to mobility during pregnancy or before insertion of epidural analgesia.
- **Blood or clotting disorder or haemaglobinopathy**
  Significance: This may be affected by the pregnancy, could lead to previous miscarriage or have an effect on clotting during pregnancy. Will need specialist referral.

Continued

Box 3.1 Health history *(Continued)*

- **Blood transfusion**
  Significance: May have developed antibodies in response to previous transfusion.
- **Cancer**
  Significance: May need close assessment due to potential of cancer regrowth or psychological need. Will need specialist referral.
- **Cardiac problems**
  Significance: Increased circulatory volume in pregnancy could compromise cardiopulmonary system. Will require specialist referral.
- **Cervical smear**
  Significance: To establish if there have been any previous abnormalities of cells.
- **Diabetes**
  Significance: Will need antenatal care coordinated between medical and obstetric team. Diabetes is associated with both maternal and neonatal morbidity (NICE 2015).
- **Epilepsy/neurological conditions**
  Significance: Small teratogenic risk from anticonvulsant therapy. Will need specialist referral to ensure drug therapy is appropriate (Kinney & Morrow 2016).
- **Exposure to toxic substances**
  Significance: May have a teratogenic effect on the fetus.
- **Female circumcision**
  Significance: May have an impact on labour and birth and emotional wellbeing. Legal requirement to report. Will need referral.
- **Fertility problems**
  Significance: May require more frequent attendance at antenatal clinic for reassurance and support.
- **Folic acid**
  Significance: 0.4 mg folic acid daily pre-conceptually and during pregnancy in the first trimester recommended to reduce the risk of neural tube defects by 75% (MRC vitamin study research group 1991).
- **Gastrointestinal problems**
  Significance: May have an impact on absorption of nutrients and general health. Will need referral.
- **Genital infections** (e.g. chlamydia, herpes)
  Significance: May return during pregnancy and affect labour. Ascending infection may result in premature labour and/or neonatal morbidity.
- **High blood pressure**
  Significance: More likely to develop pre-eclampsia; therefore need additional monitoring in pregnancy and specialist referral.
- **Incontinence (urinary/faecal)**
  Significance: May become worse in pregnancy. May need psychological support and specialist referral, especially postnatal.
- **Infections**
  Significance: If had previous serious infections or recent infections, these may have an impact on maternal or fetal morbidity.
- **Inherited disorders**
  Significance: May have an impact on fetal morbidity.

Box 3.1 Health history *(Continued)*

- **Liver disease or hepatitis**
  Significance: Cholestasis may worsen during pregnancy in women with primary biliary cirrhosis. May affect blood clotting. Will need specialist referral.
- **Migraine or severe headache**
  Significance: May become better or more intense in pregnancy.
- **Musculoskeletal problems**
  Significance: Mobility may become worse in pregnancy. Will need specialist referral.
- **Renal problems**
  Significance: Effect of progesterone in pregnancy leads to convolution of ureters, urinary stasis and thus increased potential for urinary tract infection (UTI). UTI linked with increased risk of premature labour.
- **Respiratory disease**
  Significance: Need careful assessment before the use of inhalational analgesia or surgery. Previous or active tuberculosis in pregnant women should be referred for appropriate assessment and treatment.
- **Thrombosis**
  Significance: Need prophylactic anticoagulation therapy during pregnancy and special monitoring.
- **Thyroid and endocrine conditions**
  Significance: May affect fetal morbidity. Will need specialist referral and monitoring.
- **Medication taken in last 6 months**
  Significance: To establish if there are any other conditions not identified or if women have taken any substances or over-the-counter therapies that may have an impact on fetal morbidity.
- **Vaginal bleeding in this pregnancy**
  Significance: To establish if there have been any concerns about this pregnancy before the booking appointment.

Current medical history

Women with an underlying medical disorder may become pregnant. Often, women confirm their pregnancy with their GP first; hence the woman's medical condition is already known. For example, if the woman has diabetes, the GP would refer the woman directly to a clinic that caters to pregnant women with medical conditions, or she has already been receiving preconception care. These clinics have different names, such as 'joint care clinic', where arrangements are made for both the medical team and the obstetric team to see the woman at the same time. Thus care is planned and coordinated to meet the needs of the pregnant woman in the light of her underlying medical condition. Individual maternity services may have alternative systems in place to support the care of local women.

The midwife needs to ascertain the woman's current health status to identify any potential problem that might affect either the woman's or the baby's health. Normal health is a highly subjective concept. For example, a woman who usually uses her asthma inhaler four times a day might consider her health to be very good if she has only needed to use it twice a day for the last week. Thus a question such as, 'Are you normally well?' might elicit a positive response. An alternative might be: 'Tell me about your general health. Are you currently receiving treatment for anything?' It is important to note any medication currently taken (prescribed, illegal or over the counter) to ensure that nothing is being taken that could potentially harm the developing fetus. It is also important at this point to document any known allergies to drugs or other substances. If the woman is less than 12 weeks pregnant the midwife should recommend that she takes folic acid, 400 micrograms daily, to reduce the risk of the baby having a neural tube defect.

Screening for infections

The National Institute for Health and Care Excellence recommends that women aged under 25 years should be informed at the first appointment of the high prevalence of chlamydia in their age group. They should be directed to local screening services (NICE 2008, 2017), but that chlamydia screening should not form part of routine antenatal care. It is also highlighted by NICE (2008, 2017) that all women should be offered screening for asymptomatic bacteriuria via a midstream urine sample, as early treatment reduces the risk of pyelonephritis. NICE does not recommend that women be screened routinely for beta haemolytic streptococcus. If they are known to have had a previous infection, local policy should be followed.

Activity

Find out about the implications for the unborn baby of being infected with beta haemolytic streptococcus. Identify five drugs that may have a teratogenic effect. Describe five jobs which might be hazardous during pregnancy and explain why.

Social history

The woman experiences her pregnancy within a social context. This environment may affect the health of both the woman and her baby. There are many issues to consider, including social support and financial and housing difficulties. The midwife will need to recognize potential problems and refer the woman to appropriate agencies for specialist help if needed. The following issues are of particular concern:

- **Smoking**: It is widely acknowledged that smoking in pregnancy has significant sequelae for the developing fetus, the mother and the child (Department of Health 2017). Women who smoke expect health professionals to raise the issue, and failure to do so may result in the woman concluding that the professional does not see smoking as an important issue. There are many schemes and initiatives designed to help pregnant smokers quit the habit. National guidance is that midwives should offer a carbon monoxide test and then refer all smokers to a stop smoking service (NICE 2010).

- **Alcohol:** The midwife documents the number of units of alcohol consumed by the woman each week. This provides the opportunity to answer any questions that the issue of alcohol consumption raises and to provide general guidance. Excessive alcohol consumption can potentially lead to fetal alcohol syndrome, resulting in a range of physical and mental sequelae. The level of safe drinking for pregnant women remains a controversial issue. The current guidance of the chief medical officer in the UK is to abstain during pregnancy (Department of Health 2016), though no more than one or two units, once or twice a week, may be safe (Mamluk et al 2017).

- **Drug use:** Questions may be asked related to different forms of recreational drug use, including cannabis, gas or glue and injectables. Use of such drugs puts the woman and her baby at risk of morbidity as well as a high risk of infection and may require further screening. She may then be referred to a midwife specialist in the care of women drug users.

- **Domestic abuse:** According to a UK study (Salmon et al 2015) most women do not object to being asked by their midwife about domestic abuse, including those who have reported exposure to violence. It is important that the midwife has received education about the issues surrounding domestic violence and that local guidance supports her actions when abuse is disclosed.

- **Diverse cultures:** A midwife should always be aware that the woman in front of her may be a refugee or seeking asylum (NICE 2012). In some areas a question about her status is always asked to avoid any assumptions. She may have experienced trauma in her previous circumstances such as war, abuse or female genital mutilation (FGM), and these will have affected her wellbeing. There should be awareness of the need for careful and sensitive questioning, especially when using translation services, and referral to appropriate agencies for support.

Activity

Is the first encounter with a midwife the best time to ask questions on these topics? Is this the only time? Find out the legal requirements for health professionals in relation to identifying and reporting FGM.

Family history

Again, this section in the National Maternity Records encourages the woman to identify for herself any relevant family history, including diabetes, sickle cell anaemia, thalassaemia, learning disabilities, congenital abnormalities and consanguinity. However, the midwife may need to ask for further information if a particular response has the potential to affect the future plan of care. It is important to identify conditions that may have relevance to this pregnancy either in terms of the need for specialist referral or to allay unwarranted fears.

Previous obstetric history

It is important to pay particular attention to a woman's previous experiences. These memories may contribute to how she feels about the forthcoming birth of this baby. It may be an opportunity to clarify misconceptions and address concerns. Table 3.1 identified aspects of each birth that should be documented.

Taking an accurate previous obstetric history will help highlight factors that might warrant the woman being referred for consultant opinion. For example, women who have had a previous low birth weight baby should be closely monitored and offered serial ultrasound scans to identify potential sub-optimum growth in the pregnancy. Being aware of previous events such as emergency caesarean birth, premature labour, antepartum or postpartum haemorrhage, previous small or large baby, pre-eclampsia and

Table 3.1: Previous obstetric history

Suggested questions:			
Date of birth	Boy/girl/name	Gestation	Birthweight/centile
Health at birth	Alive and well now	Method of feeding	Where now?
Birth details	Spontaneous/induced	Vaginal/assisted	Planned/emergency CS
Anaesthesia	None/entonox	Epidural	Spinal/general
Third stage	Spontaneous/active	Retained	Postpartum haemorrhage
Perineum	Intact	Tear 1°/2°/3°	Episiotomy
Postnatal health	Well/complications	Postnatal depression	Puerperal Psychosis

gestational diabetes will enable the midwife to plan appropriate and individualized antenatal care.

> **Activity**
>
> Find out what is meant by parity. How would you describe a woman in obstetric terms who was pregnant for the third time, having had one live child and a miscarriage at 10 weeks?

Current obstetric history

It is important to assess how the woman is feeling. So much of the focus so far has been on related issues rather than this pregnancy. The midwife will ask what symptoms of pregnancy the woman has experienced and how she feels generally about being pregnant. She will also establish the first day of the woman's last menstrual period (LMP) and from this estimate the woman's expected date of delivery (EDD). See Table 3.2.

This calculation is based on a 28-day menstrual cycle. It is important that the midwife establishes what was normal for the woman: how often she bled and for how long. She will ask if the last period was a 'normal' period, as occasionally women experience a small blood loss (nidation) when the fertilized ovum (blastocyst) embeds in the endometrium. As this occurs at approximately the same time as the next period might have been anticipated, it can occasionally be incorrectly perceived as such. NICE (2008, 2017) recommends that all women are offered an ultrasound scan between 10 weeks and 13 plus 6 days to confirm the gestation of the fetus and exclude multiple pregnancy.

> **Activity**
>
> The first day of Joanna's LMP was 15/8/17. How many weeks pregnant is she now? Be sure that you can make these calculations using both a calendar and a gestation calculator (wheel). What percentage of babies are born on their EDD?

Table 3.2: Calculating expected date of delivery

First day of last menstrual period (LMP)	21/8/18
Add 1 year	21/8/19
Add 7 days	28/8/19
Take away 3 months	28/5/19
EDD	28/5/19

Table 3.3: BMI classification (WHO 2017)

Underweight	BMI <18.5
Desirable	BMI 18.5–24.9
Overweight	BMI 25.0–29.9
Obesity class I	BMI 30–34.9
Obesity class II	BMI 35–39.9
Obesity class III	BMI 40 or more

Physical characteristics

Weight is not routinely monitored throughout pregnancy (NICE 2008, 2017) by healthcare professionals (although it may be by women), but it is important to establish a baseline at the start of maternity care. It is also recommended that the body mass index (BMI), or the ratio of weight in kilogrammes to height in metres squared, is calculated as a determinant of higher weight in women (NICE 2008, 2017).

The World Health Organization (WHO 2017) has recognized a range of categories of BMI (Table 3.3). Increasing BMI is associated with gestational diabetes, hypertension, thromboembolism and anaesthetic risk, and should be calculated at booking (NICE 2008, 2017). The latest Confidential Enquiries into Maternal Deaths (Knight et al 2017) highlighted that over half of the women who died in the triennium 2013–15 were of higher weight (BMI over 25) and 34% were obese. The midwife should then follow local guidance regarding referral to a dietician for appropriate assessment and monitoring once higher BMI is diagnosed.

Age is also recorded, as extremes of the childbearing continuum are associated with adverse obstetric outcomes. A woman's age may influence the pathway of care, for example, consideration of induction of labour at 39 to 40 weeks' gestation to reduce the risk of stillbirth (Page et al 2013). Women aged over 40 years have an increased risk of pre-eclampsia, and more frequent monitoring of blood pressure and urinalysis for proteinurea throughout pregnancy should be considered (NICE 2008, 2017).

Clinical observations

The midwife will test the woman's urine for protein and take her blood pressure, both routine aspects of subsequent antenatal care (NICE 2008, 2017). A midstream specimen of urine should also be sent to the laboratory for culture to test for the presence of asymptomatic bacteriuria (NICE 2008, 2017), as treatment can prevent pylonephritis, a potentially serious kidney infection. It is also important that an abdominal palpation is undertaken at this time to pick up advancing or multiple pregnancy, as the uterus is not normally palpable above the symphysis pubis until approximately 12 weeks' gestation. Blood will also be taken to check Joanna's blood group and rhesus factor and check for anaemia, HIV and syphilis (see Chapter 7).

Assessing for appropriate care

Taking a booking history is an opportunity to undertake an appropriate assessment of the pregnancy to ensure the woman receives appropriate care. In the past it was reported that there were some cases where only midwifery-led care had been provided to women who were known to be at high risk of complications. This puts both the woman and her baby at risk, and is not in the scope of practice of a midwife. However, this may be the choice of the woman, if she has been provided with, and weighed up, the information to decide what is right for her (Byrom & Byrom 2017). *Better Births* (National Maternity Review 2016:44) highlights the need for personalized care plans created jointly by the woman and midwife that *'recognise that risk is not binary or absolute, but seeks to accommodate that risk.'*

Information giving

It is recommended that women take 10 micrograms of vitamin D each day during pregnancy (NICE 2008, 2017). Vitamin D is made by the body through exposure to sunlight and is essential for the development of healthy bones. Those who require this supplement most are:

- 'Women with darker skin (such as those of African, African–Caribbean or South Asian family origin
- Women who have limited exposure to sunlight, such as women who are housebound or confined indoors for long periods, or who cover their skin for cultural reasons.' (NICE 2008, 2017)

NICE guidelines (2008, 2017) also recommend that women receive information at booking about how the baby develops during pregnancy, nutrition and diet and exercise, including pelvic floor exercises. They also suggest that women are informed about antenatal classes, maternity benefits, and breastfeeding workshops.

Discuss place of birth

Women need to be aware of the options available about place of birth in their locality before they can make a decision about what might be best for them. Place of birth is a complicated issue, and many factors need to be considered before a fully informed decision can be made. The booking visit is an ideal opportunity to raise the issue, to let the woman know that she has a choice, but not necessarily the right time to seek a definitive decision. In some services, women are not asked to make a decision until they go into labour. In a survey of women in 2015 (Care Quality Commission 2015) just 58% felt they had been given enough information to make the choice about which place of birth was right for them. It is evident from this survey that there is inconsistency in whether women are offered birth in a midwifery-led unit or home birth, as recommended by NICE (2014, 2017).

Although many midwives freely offer choice regarding place of birth, some do not. This may be due to a range of reasons, including lack of confidence due to infrequent demand (McCourt et al 2012). Some midwives may work in a team where the other midwives would not be able to cover her clinic or visits if she is called to a home birth. Crises of low staffing levels sometimes lead units to temporarily withdraw home birth as an option.

Home birth presents the ideal scenario of one-to-one care in labour for women at low risk of complication. A woman booked for a hospital birth may be cared for by a midwife who is also looking after other women at the same time. The Birthplace Study (Birthplace in England Collaborative Group 2011) has shown that home birth is a safe option for both mother and baby, though there is a slightly increased risk of morbidity for the baby in first-time labours. However, it would be inappropriate for all women to give birth at home, as there are limited options for pharmacological methods of pain relief. Others have or develop complications either during their pregnancy or birth that preclude home birth as a suitable option, as they require the facilities of an obstetric unit and medical or surgical support. Other options are midwife-led units which are either freestanding (away from the main hospital unit) or alongside (on the premises of the main hospital unit). Births in these units have also been demonstrated to be safe and should be an option for all women (NICE 2014, 2017).

Women need to be aware of the risks and benefits of the options they choose, and although we are often quick to raise the risks associated with home birth or midwife-led care, we are seldom forthright in presenting the risks associated with birth in a hospital environment.

Activity

Find out what options are available for birth for women in your locality. List the advantages and disadvantages that you perceive might be associated with home, midwife-led unit and hospital birth. What obstetric complications might result in a woman being advised to give birth in hospital?

Discuss screening

A definition of screening in health contexts is:

> The process of identifying healthy people who may be at increased risk of disease or condition. The screening provider then offers information, further tests and treatment. This is to reduce associated risks or complications.

> (Public Health England 2013)

Activity

Think about all the aspects of health included in the questions for the woman in this chapter. Apply the previous definition and consider how many of these may be classed as 'screening'.

The history-taking interview is often the time when women are given information about the options available to them regarding antenatal screening for fetal abnormality. They may have already heard about some of the tests through a relative or friends. However, women need to make choices that are right for them as individuals and may require support and guidance about the potential risks and benefits of the test on offer. The midwife needs to be able to present the facts without prejudice or personal influence and enable 'women to make informed choices about their health and health care' (NMC 2017:5).

The range of tests available varies from locality to locality and may change as new tests become available. Keeping up to date with all the tests on offer presents a challenge to midwives, as they need to know what the test involves, when it is performed, how it is obtained and what the results mean. They also have to be able to translate this into meaningful information for women of all cultures and backgrounds. Keeping abreast of changes in clinical practice and applying evidence are part of a midwife's professional responsibility (NMC 2017). All women have the right to this information. If a test can only be undertaken through a private company and requires payment, it is not for the midwife to decide if a woman of low socio-economic status should have it or not. Women may face dilemmas about the choices they make, but they will not be able to address them unless they know that they exist. Midwives may have their assumptions challenged with regard to who will benefit from information (Kirkham et al 2002). See Chapter 8 for information about the screening tests available.

Activity

Find out what screening tests are offered for women who book at the trust where you work. Are they offered to all women or just to women in particular categories?

Plan appropriate antenatal care

The midwife has collected a wealth of information about the woman's previous and current health status. National guidance and local policy will suggest the course of action for women identified with complications, who should be their lead professional and how often they should be seen. However, women should at all times be treated as individuals, and midwives should aim to meet these needs (NHS England 2016; Scottish Gov 2017). National guidance from the NICE (2008, 2017) recommends 10 appointments for nulliparous women and 7 for parous women. Women will continue to need support from their community-based midwife, even if they are having specialist consultant care. The plan of action should be discussed and agreed with the woman and then documented in her maternity records.

REFLECTION ON THE TRIGGER SCENARIO

Look back on the trigger scenario.

Joanna is in the first trimester of her first pregnancy. She bought a pregnancy test at home and went to see her general practitioner (GP), who gave her some general advice about what she should and should not be eating. Aware of her previous medical history, the GP told Joanna to go to the reception desk and make an appointment for the clinic of the community midwife to undertake the 'booking'. A week later she received a package of information and a letter from the midwife confirming the appointment time and asking Joanna to produce a specimen of urine on the day of the visit.

This scenario presents a traditional model of care whereby the woman goes to her family doctor first to confirm her pregnancy before accessing midwifery care. As the GP has access to her medical notes, she deems her to be 'low risk' and therefore refers her to the community midwife for her booking history. Now that you are familiar with the purpose and content of the booking visit, you should have insight into how the scenario reflects current practice. The jigsaw model will now be used to explore the trigger scenario in more depth.

Effective communication

Effective verbal and non-verbal communication is essential in the provision of effective maternity care. Joanna has been to see her GP, who also gave her information about healthy eating in pregnancy. Questions that arise from the scenario might include the following: Did the GP explain the rationale behind the advice she gave? Was the information backed up by written information? Was written information supported by a verbal explanation? What methods of communication are there between the receptionist and the midwife, and how long does it take for the midwife to become alert to a new pregnancy? What information did Joanna receive through the post? Would it be referred to during the booking interview?

Woman-centred care

Providing personalized care centred around the woman's individual circumstances is central to current maternity policy. Questions that arise from the scenario might include the following: Did the GP offer Joanna any options for care? Was there time during the consultation with the GP for Joanna to ask specific questions? Were any specific risk factors associated with Joanna's medical or family history that made her at risk in any way? Was the letter from her midwife personal to Joanna's circumstances or was it routine?

Using best evidence

Providing women with information that is based on best evidence enables them to make informed decisions and take an active role in their care. Questions that arise from the scenario might include the following: Was the GP aware of the latest guidance from NICE? How is this information disseminated to all health professionals involved in maternity care? Are national guidelines discussed at a local level and previous care pathways amended in their light? What is the evidence about the most appropriate times to give women information? Why is it important to detect asymptomatic bacteriuria? Can women choose a pathway of care that is outside of national guidance?

Professional and legal issues

Midwives must practice within a professional and legal framework to ensure that they protect the women they care for from potential harm and maintain high standards of care. Questions that arise from the scenario might include the following: Did the GP ask Joanna's consent to refer her to the community midwife? Can the midwife ask the practice nurse to undertake the booking visit? What must the midwife do if she detects an abnormality in Joanna's pregnancy? How is the midwife keeping up to date with changes in antenatal care?

Team working

Joanna has already been in contact with four people in relation to her pregnancy: the pharmacist who sold her folic acid, the receptionist who made her GP appointment and who referred her to the midwife, the GP and the midwife by letter. Questions that arise from the scenario might include the following: How can team working in primary care be enhanced? What might the consequences be for Joanna if the midwife did not receive her referral? What might the consequences be for the midwife? Has the GP provided relevant information to the midwife about Joanna's past and current health status? What mechanisms are there for the community midwife to continue to keep the GP informed of her progress?

Clinical dexterity

Part of the booking visit includes blood pressure measurement, urinalysis and venepuncture. All of these clinical observations and procedures require clinical dexterity, confidence and competence. Questions that arise from the scenario might include the following: How did the midwife learn how to take blood, and how was this assessed? When would the midwife undertake a dip test for urinalysis versus an automated test? What equipment does the midwife use to take a woman's blood pressure in the home? How does this differ from the equipment the GP might use? What would the midwife do if she could not get a blood sample from Joanna after two attempts?

Models of care

There are many models of care, ranging from midwife-led to consultant-led antenatal care. The midwife is responsible for informing women of their options and enabling them to choose the most appropriate option for their individual circumstances. It is not stated in the scenario how this was discussed with Joanna. Questions that arise from the scenario might include the following: What is the full range of options for antenatal care in your locality? What factors influence the model of care chosen? How might the model of care chosen influence the outcome of pregnancy?

Safe environment

It is essential that the midwife takes appropriate precautionary measures when providing clinical care to women. These include ensuring that the environment does not pose a risk to either the woman or herself and following clinical procedures with care. Questions that arise from the scenario might include the following: Did the midwife wear gloves to take blood from Joanna? How did the midwife dispose of the urine dipstick? When did the midwife wash her hands? How did the midwife dispose of the needle used for venepuncture? How did the midwife check Joanna's personal details for labelling the specimens?

Promotes health

When the woman contacts the GP or midwife at the beginning of pregnancy, it provides her carers with an ideal opportunity to give her information to enable her to make informed healthcare choices. Joanna had already had input from the GP about healthy eating and then information from the midwife through the post before the booking visit. Questions that arise from the scenario might include the following: What information should the woman receive before her booking history is taken? What advice can the midwife give at booking that will promote Joanna's health during the pregnancy and throughout motherhood? What facilities are there where you work to support a pregnant woman who wishes to stop smoking?

Further scenarios

The following scenarios enable you to consider how specific situations influence the care the midwife provides. Use the jigsaw model to explore the issues raised in each scenario.

SCENARIO 1

Mary is a 43-year-old mother of two grown children. She is recently divorced and is seeing a man she does not intend staying with. She is unsure about whether to continue with her pregnancy and goes to the GP for advice. He refers her to the community midwife for a home booking visit.

Practice point

At all times midwives need to be professional and provide a duty of care to women. The midwife will need to be sensitive in this situation and prepared to listen to the woman's concerns. However, a midwife is not a trained counsellor and may need to refer her to others to help with the decision-making process.

Further questions specific to Scenario 1 include:

1. Has the GP asked Mary if she wants to continue with the pregnancy?
2. How would you tactfully approach this issue?
3. Is a home booking appropriate in these circumstances?
4. What systems are in place to offer choice to women regarding where the booking interview takes place?
5. What advice and information might the midwife offer Mary?
6. How do you feel about termination of pregnancy in these circumstances?

SCENARIO 2

Jessica is 6 weeks pregnant and keen to have a home birth. She makes an appointment directly with the midwife to discuss how to go about this.

Practice point

Women are to be encouraged to have midwives as the first point of contact, as this can help in building relationships and promoting health in early pregnancy.

Further questions specific to Scenario 2 include:

1. Is there an optimum time to discuss place of birth?
2. How can the midwife support Jessica in her aspirations?
3. Are there any circumstances where a midwife should recommend that Jessica have a hospital birth?
4. Should parity influence the decision in any way?
5. What advice can the midwife offer Jessica to help her achieve her dream?

Conclusion

The booking history presents a unique opportunity for the woman and midwife to form a relationship and develop mutual respect. It may be the first time that the woman has come across a midwife, and she may be unclear about the midwife's role and what to expect from antenatal care. Ideally she will come away feeling that she has met someone who is competent and caring and with whom she can discuss her hopes and fears.

Resources
Department of Health
https://www.gov.uk/government/organisations/department-of-health
Female Genital Mutilation
http://www.dofeve.org/about-fgm.html

http://forwarduk.org.uk/key-issues/fgm/
Fetal alcohol syndrome - NOFAS charity
http://www.nofas-uk.org/
Health Scotland
http://www.gov.scot/Topics/Health
Healthy Start
https://www.healthystart.nhs.uk/
Mental Health in Pregnancy
http://www.rcpsych.ac.uk/expertadvice/problems/mentalhealthinpregnancy.aspx
Nutrition in Pregnancy
https://www.nutrition.org.uk/healthyliving/nutritionforpregnancy.html
Stopping Smoking
https://www.nhs.uk/smokefree
Public Health England
https://www.gov.uk/government/organisations/public-health-england

References

Birthplace in England Collaborative Group, Brocklehurst, P., Hardy, P., et al., 2011. Perinatal and maternal outcomes by planned place of birth for healthy women with low risk pregnancies: the Birthplace in England national prospective cohort study. Br. Med. J. 2011, 343.

Brown, H.C., Smith, H.J., Mori, R., Norma, H., 2015. Giving women their own case notes to carry during pregnancy. Cochrane Database Syst. Rev. 2015. (10), Art. No.: CD002856, doi:10.1002/14651858.CD002856.pub3.

Byrom, S., Byrom, A., 2017. Choice, childbearing and maternity care: the choice agenda and place of birth. In: MacDonald, S., Johnson, G. (Eds.), Mayes Midwifery Elsevier. London.

Cambridge, J., 2012. Language barriers: my interpretation. RCM Midwives J. 15 (3), 29.

Care Quality Commission, 2015. 2015 survey of women's experiences of maternity care. Available from: http://www.cqc.org.uk/sites/default/files/20151215b_mat15_statistical_release.pdf.

Department of Health, 2016. UK Chief Medical Officers' Alcohol Guidelines Review. http://www.drugsandalcohol.ie/25010/1/CMO_UK_Alcohol_guidelines_review_summary.pdf.

Department of Health, 2017. Towards a Smokefree Generation. A Tobacco Control Plan for England. Available at: https://www.gov.uk/government/uploads/system/uploads/attachment_data/file/630217/Towards_a_Smoke_free_Generation_-_A_Tobacco_Control_Plan_for_England_2017-2022__2_.pdf. (Accessed 29 September 2017).

Hall, J., Collins, B., Ireland, J., Hundley, V., 2016. The Human Rights & Dignity Experience of Disabled Women during Pregnancy, Childbirth and Early Parenting. Available from: http://www.birthrights.org.uk/wordpress/wp-content/uploads/2016/09/Interim-Report-Dignity-Experience-Disabled-Women.pdf.

Kinney, M.O., Morrow, J., 2016. Epilepsy in pregnancy. Available from: http://www.bmj.com/content/353/bmj.i2880.

Kirkham, M., Stapleton, H., Curtis, P., Thomas, G., 2002. Stereotyping as a professional defence mechanism. Br. J. Midwifery 10 (9), 549–552.

Knight, M., Nair, M., Tuffnell, D., et al. (Eds.), on behalf of MBRRACE-UK, 2017. Saving Lives, Improving Mothers' Care - Lessons learned to inform maternity care from the UK and Ireland Confidential Enquiries into Maternal Deaths and Morbidity 2013–15. National Perinatal Epidemiology Unit, University of Oxford, Oxford. https://www.npeu.ox.ac.uk/downloads/files/mbrrace-uk/reports/MBRRACE-UK%20Maternal%20Report%202017%20-%20 Web.pdf.

Locatis, C., Williamson, D., Gould-Kabler, C., et al., 2010. Comparing In-Person, Video, and Telephonic Medical Interpretation. J. Gen. Intern. Med. 25 (4), 345–350. http://doi.org/10.1007/s11606-009-1236-x.

Mamluk, L., Edwards, H.B., Savović, J., et al., 2017. Low alcohol consumption and pregnancy and childhood outcomes: time to change guidelines indicating apparently 'safe' levels of alcohol during pregnancy? A systematic review and meta-analyses. BMJ Open 7, e015410. doi:10.1136/bmjopen-2016-015410.

McCourt, C., 2006. Supporting choice and control? Communication and interaction between midwives and women at the antenatal booking visit. Soc. Sci. Med. 62 (6), 1307–1318.

McCourt, C., Rayment, J., Rance, S., Sandall, J., 2012. Organisational strategies and midwives' readiness to provide care for out of hospital births: An analysis from the birthplace organisational case studies. Midwifery 28 (5), 636–645. doi:10.1016/j.midw.2012.07.004.

Methven, E., 1989. Recording an obstetric history or relating to pregnant women? A study of the antenatal booking interview. In: Robinson, S., Thomson, A.M. (Eds.), Midwives, Research and Childbirth, vol. I. Chapman and Hall, London.

MRC vitamin study research group, 1991. Prevention of neural tube defects: results of the medical research council research council vitamin study. Lancet 338 (8760), 131–137.

NHS England, 2016. National Maternity Service Review. Better Births, Improving outcomes of maternity services in England 5 year forward view for the maternity services. DH, London.

NICE, 2008, 2017. Antenatal Care for uncomplicated pregnancies clinical guideline. https://www.nice.org.uk/guidance/cg62.

NICE, 2010. Smoking: stopping in pregnancy and after childbirth. https://www.nice.org.uk/guidance/ph26.

NICE, 2012. Pregnancy and complex social factors: a model for service provision for pregnant women with complex social factors. https://www.nice.org.uk/guidance/CG110/chapter/1-Guidance#pregnant-women-who-are-recent-migrants-asylum-seekers-or-refugees-or-who-have-difficulty-reading.

NICE, 2014, 2017. Intrapartum care for healthy women and babies. https://www.nice.org.uk/guidance/cg190/chapter/Recommendations#place-of-birth.

NICE, 2015. Diabetes in pregnancy: management from preconception to the postnatal period https://www.nice.org.uk/guidance/ng3/chapter/Introduction.

Nursing and Midwifery Council, 2015. The Code: Professional standards of practice and behaviour for nurses and midwives. https://www.nmc.org.uk/globalassets/sitedocuments/nmc-publications/nmc-code.pdf.

Nursing and Midwifery Council, 2017. Standards for competence for registered midwives. https://www.nmc.org.uk/globalassets/sitedocuments/standards/nmc-standards-for-competence-for-registered-midwives.pdf.

Page, J., Snowden, J., Cheng, Y., et al., 2013. The Risk of Stillbirth and Infant Death by Each Additional Week of Expectant Management Stratified by Maternal Age. Am. J. Obstet. Gynecol. 209 (4), 375.e1–75.e7. Web.

Public Health England, 2013. NHS Population screening explained. https://www.gov.uk/guidance/nhs-population-screening-explained.

RCM, 2011. High Quality Maternity care. Available from: https://www.rcm.org.uk/sites/default/files/High%20Quality%20Midwifery%20Care%20Final.pdf.

Robinson, M., 2002. Communication and health in a multi-ethnic society. Policy Press, Bristol.

Rungapadiachy, D.M., 1999. Interpersonal communication and psychology for the health care professional: Theory and practice. Butterworth-Heinemann, Oxford.

Salmon, D., Baird, K.M., White, P., 2015. Women's views and experiences of antenatal enquiry for domestic abuse during pregnancy. Health Expect. 18 (5), 867–878. doi:10.1111/hex.12060.

Scottish Gov, 2017. The best start - a five year forward plan for maternity and neonatal care in Scotland. Available from: http://www.gov.scot/Resource/0051/00513175.pdf.

World Health Organization, 2017. BMI classification. http://www.who.int/bmi/index.jsp?introPage=intro_3.html.

CHAPTER 4

Health in pregnancy

TRIGGER SCENARIO

Joanna is now 20 weeks pregnant. She has been well, although rather nauseous at times, but this is now less frequent. She gave up smoking 3 weeks ago and is now beginning to struggle. She even got to the stage where she took one of Louis's cigarettes from the packet and searched through the kitchen drawer to find a lighter that worked. She was interrupted by an interesting text message and then managed to gather her willpower to put the cigarette back in its packet.

Introduction

Pregnancy is not an illness, but a time of changing physiology and great anticipation. This chapter will focus on factors that impact on both the woman's health and that of her developing baby. Issues that relate specifically to emotional wellbeing and mental health will be considered in Chapter 6.

Many sources of information are available for women regarding achieving a healthy pregnancy. These are produced by government agencies, commercial businesses, local trusts, user and support groups and professional bodies. Some women experience very few problems in relation to their health, have a spontaneous labour and give birth to a healthy baby without making any conscious changes to their usual way of life. However, many women seek and require advice about the physical and emotional changes they experience and look to the midwife for support and the provision of effective information.

Activity

Find out what information is available for women regarding health in pregnancy in your locality. Who produces it? Is it clear and easy to understand? Is it available in a range of different languages? How many UK websites offer information for pregnant women?

Health in pregnancy

One rationale for achieving a healthy lifestyle during pregnancy is to maximize the likelihood of having a healthy baby and to avoid inadvertently harming the baby by being unaware of potentially hazardous behaviour. Women need information so that they can make decisions about how they alter or adapt their lifestyle. Health promotion in pregnancy is also to help the woman make choices that will affect her long-term wellbeing and that of her family. It is not currently a criminal offence in the United Kingdom for a woman to potentially put her baby at risk, for example, by smoking or drinking alcohol during pregnancy, but this has become the situation in other countries. However, it is part of the midwife's role to advise women during pregnancy and offer health counselling and education (International Confederation of Midwives (ICM) 2017). To fail to inform women of known potential risks to their or their baby's health would be to breach her duty of care. The midwife therefore needs to have a working knowledge of how women can optimize women's health, for the benefit of both their own and their baby's wellbeing.

Activity

Find out why pregnant women should avoid pregnant ewes and newborn lambs. Why should pregnant women wear gloves when gardening or changing cat litter? How should cooked and uncooked meats be stored in the refrigerator?

Diet

The issue of what pregnant women eat has provided much food for thought over the years. Aspects of debate include the quantity and quality of food and pregnancy-associated changes to women's dietary intake. It has been reported that maternal nutrition during pregnancy may have a significant impact on future adult health (Bayol et al 2008; Shalini et al 2015).

Activity

In an ideal world a woman should enter pregnancy in a state of optimum health.

Find out about the principles of preconception care for both women and their partners. What is the role of the midwife in preconception care?

Quantity

Although it is not part of general antenatal care to weigh women every time they attend clinic (National Institute for Health and Care Excellence (NICE) 2008, 2017), many women do keep an eye on their own weight gain. There is a wide range of weight gain associated with a normal outcome and a wide range of thoughts about what should be 'average'. Definitive guidance on how much weight a woman with normal body mass index (BMI) should put on during pregnancy is scarce: the U.S. Institute of Medicine suggests approximately 11 to 16 kilograms as appropriate (Institute of Medicine 2009). UK guidance suggests that the pregnant woman does not need any extra calories until the final 3 months, when her intake should increase by 200 kcal daily (NICE 2010a). Her diet should be balanced (see The Eatwell Guide, Public Health England 2016) with increased thiamine; riboflavin; folate; vitamins A, C and D; calcium; selenium; iodine; and omega-3 and -6 fatty acids (Jewell 2017).

Dietary restriction in pregnancy can result in reduction in birth weight and preterm birth and some long-term effects on metabolism (Grieger & Clifton 2015). The NICE guidance on improving nutrition for pregnant and breastfeeding mothers (NICE 2008, 2014) highlights the prevalence of malnutrition, particularly in low-income households, with one-fifth of adults having small meals or skipping them altogether. Women with low incomes are eligible for Healthy Start vouchers to enable them to buy fruit and vegetables (https://www.healthystart.nhs.uk/). A systematic review (Ota et al 2015) found that antenatal nutritional education with the aim of increasing energy and protein intake in the general obstetric population appears to be effective in reducing:

> the risk of preterm birth, low birthweight, increasing head circumference at birth, increasing birthweight among undernourished women, and increasing protein intake resulted in both maternal weight gain and increased birth weight with a subsequent decrease in small for gestational age infants and lower perinatal mortality.

Obesity in pregnancy is associated with increased obstetric risk, including gestational diabetes, hypertension, operative intervention, anaesthetic complications, prolonged labour and shoulder dystocia (Ovesen et al 2011). There is also evidence that maternal obesity is associated with an increased risk of fetal abnormality (Rankin et al 2010). The recent Confidential Enquiries into Maternal Deaths (Knight et al 2017) highlighted that over half of the women who died in the triennium 2013–15 were of higher weight (BMI over 25) and 34% were obese. Although women are often advised not to lose weight in pregnancy (NICE 2010a), this may be a time when they are receptive to nutritional advice (Richens 2008). A systematic review of the benefits of a low-glycaemic diet in pregnancy to reduce the risks of gestational diabetes mellitus (Tieu et al 2017) concluded that although the results suggested this to be beneficial, the evidence was not strong enough to be conclusive. Claesson et al (2008) report on a case-control intervention study of motivational talks and aquarobic exercise classes for women of higher weight. Although the intervention was not associated with any difference between the groups for obstetric variables, the intervention group had significantly less weight gain during pregnancy than the control group. Women with a BMI over 30 kg/m^2 should be referred for consultant care and screened for diabetes (NICE 2008, 2017). Those women with a BMI over 35 kg/m^2 should be advised to take aspirin therapy to mitigate their increased risk of pre-eclampsia (NICE 2010, 2011).

Quality

Women are faced with an increasing range of foods that they are advised not to eat when pregnant because of the potential risk to the developing fetus. Many supplements are available over the counter for women considering pregnancy or who are currently pregnant.

Soft cheese, unpasteurized dairy products and pâté

These foods are associated with the bacteria known as *Listeria monocytogenes*. All fruit and vegetables should be washed before eating, as the bacteria is found in soil. The bacteria are killed by heat, and women should be advised to ensure that all meats are cooked thoroughly and that takeaway food is eaten piping hot (NICE 2008, 2017). The infection may present as flu-like symptoms in the pregnant woman and can be transferred to the fetus via the placenta or during birth. When contracted before birth, the baby may develop septicaemia, with an associated mortality rate of 20% to 30%, although this is reduced if the infection is confirmed and antibiotic therapy is given (Janakiraman 2008). Offensive liquor and placental cysts may alert the midwife to suspect infection, initiating investigation, diagnosis and appropriate treatment.

Liver (vitamin A)

Although pregnant women do need small amounts of this vitamin, found in liver, it should not be consumed in large amounts or taken in dietary supplements due to the teratogenic effects of toxicity (NICE 2008, 2017).

Swordfish, marlin and shark

These fish should not be eaten due to their high methyl mercury content, which could affect the nervous system of the developing fetus (First Steps

Nutrition 2017). There is evidence to suggest that women who consume a diet low in seafood are more at risk of premature labour (Klebanoff et al 2011; Olsen & Secher 2002).

Suggested supplements in pregnancy

Folic acid and iron

It is recommended that women have a diet rich in folic acid and take folic acid supplementation before conception and up to the twelfth week of pregnancy to reduce the risk of having a baby with a neural tube defect (Wald et al 1991). The recommended dose is 400 micrograms daily (NICE 2008, 2017). Folic acid is also important for the formation of red blood cells, and folic acid–rich foods include sprouts, asparagus, peas, broccoli, oranges and bananas (First Steps Nutrition 2017). Women should also ensure that their diet is rich in iron, which is necessary for the production of red blood cells. Iron-rich foods include red meat, fortified cereals, grains and pulses and leafy green vegetables (First Steps Nutrition 2017). There is no evidence that routine iron supplementation has any benefit for the health outcomes of either mother or baby (Peña-Rosas et al 2015), and they are not recommended for all women in antenatal care (NICE 2008, 2017).

Vitamin D

It is recommended that women take 10 micrograms of vitamin D each day during pregnancy (NICE 2008, 2017). Vitamin D helps regulate the amount of calcium and phosphate in the body, which are required for the formation of bones and teeth. Vitamin D is particularly important for women with darker skin and those not often exposed to sunlight, such as women who do not or are unable to go out of the house much or who cover their skin for cultural reasons.

Box 4.1 highlights physical changes that take place through pregnancy that may affect dietary intake.

Activity

Find out what is meant by hyperemesis gravidarum. What is the incidence and who is most at risk? How would the midwife recognize this condition? What is the treatment?

Salt

A systematic review of the evidence related to reducing salt intake in pregnancy with a view to preventing or reducing the risk of pre-eclampsia did not show any evidence of benefit to mother or baby (Duley et al 2005). It is, however, a recommendation that adults do not consume more than

Box 4.1 Changes during pregnancy affecting dietary intake

Nausea and vomiting

Affects 80% of pregnant women; exacerbated by fatigue; some symptoms relieved by small, frequent, high-carbohydrate meals, ginger, acupressure at P6 on the wrist or through the use of antihistamines (NICE 2008, 2017). For up to 2% of women vomiting is a serious condition called *hyperemesis gravidarum* (McCarthy et al 2014).

Increased appetite and thirst

Experienced by more than 50% of women (Coad & Dunstall 2011). Capacity of the stomach reduced in late pregnancy due to displacement by gravid uterus.

Cravings

Women sometimes have cravings for unusual food combinations during pregnancy, and these are usually harmless. Alternatively, women may develop a dislike for foods and drinks normally enjoyed, such as tea and coffee. This may be exacerbated by a metallic taste in the mouth. Consuming or craving substances that have no nutritional food value is known as *pica*.

Increased salivation

The term *ptyalism* refers to the experience of excess saliva in the mouth, although there is no evidence to confirm excess production, but rather that swallowing saliva induces nausea in some women, resulting in a tendency for it to collect in the mouth (Thaxter Nesbeth et al 2016).

Indigestion

Increased progesterone levels lead to impaired competence of the cardiac sphincter of the stomach. Reflux acid causes epigastric pain exacerbated by large or spicy meals. Maintaining an upright posture can help prevent gastric reflux. Antacids are sometimes required to alleviate symptoms (NICE 2008, 2017).

Constipation

Relaxation of smooth muscle of gastrointestinal tract due to progesterone. Slower passage of food; increased absorption of water. Constipation may be exacerbated by some oral iron therapy. Need to increase fibre content of diet (e.g. cereals, fresh fruit and vegetables). A systematic review of interventions for treating constipation in pregnancy concluded that the use of fibre supplements would increase stool frequency (Rungsiprakarn et al 2015). They also established that bowel stimulants were more effective than bulking agents, but were more likely to lead to abdominal pain and diarrhoea. Haemorrhoids may compound the problem.

6 grams of salt daily to reduce the risk of hypertension and associated vascular disease (First Steps Nutrition Trust 2017).

Caffeine

It is recommended (Care study group 2008) that women do not consume more than 200 mg of caffeine per day, as excessive intake has been linked to low birth weight (Chen et al 2014). There is some evidence to show that even 100 mg may have an impact for some women (Rhee et al 2015). It is advisable to consider carefully the amount of caffeine consumed in any drink during pregnancy.

Lifestyle choices

Alcohol

Midwives need to find ways to explore women's alcohol consumption in a sensitive, non-judgemental way, as it is thought that under-reporting is widespread (Royal College of Obstetrics and Gynaecology (RCOG) 2006). A consistently high consumption of alcohol is linked with a series of characteristics that together are known as *fetal alcohol syndrome (FAS)*.

Activity

FAS manifests in a number of ways. Access the charity site the National Organisation for Foetal Alcohol Syndrome (NOFAS) http://www.nofas-uk .org/?cat=14 and look at the list of characteristics. Consider how you would discuss alcohol consumption with women in pregnancy.

Binge drinking has been highlighted as being particularly harmful (NICE 2008, 2017). It is recommended that women abstain from drinking alcohol throughout pregnancy; however, if women do continue to drink, consumption should not exceed one to two measures once or twice a week (Department of Health 2016).

Smoking

Both professionals and members of the public are now well aware that smoking is hazardous to extra-uterine and intra-uterine health. Box 4.2 lists some of the potential effects of smoking in pregnancy. However, despite this knowledge, many pregnant women and their partners continue to smoke. Many women who smoke are living in challenging circumstances and find it very difficult to give up. They need support to quit, and many local initiatives are designed to provide advice and encouragement. Access to services depends on the midwife identifying the need for support and using her interpersonal skills to discuss the topic in a non-judgemental manner. The midwife needs to be aware of her own feelings with regard to women who smoke. If she alienates the woman when she asks the first question, 'Do you smoke?' either by the tone of her voice or the look on her face, it may be difficult to repair the damage. It is important not to push information on a woman who does not want to give up smoking; however, it is prudent to assess if the woman is aware of the dangers to

Box 4.2 List of potential impacts of smoking tobacco in pregnancy (RCOG 2015a)

- Miscarriage
- Ectopic pregnancy
- Stillbirth or dying shortly after birth – one-third of all deaths in the womb or shortly after birth are thought to be caused by smoking
- Baby born with abnormalities – face defects, such as cleft lip and palate, are more common because smoking affects the way a baby develops
- Poor growth of baby – poor health, potentially long term
- Abruption of the placenta
- Preterm birth
- Increased risk of:
  - Sudden infant death syndrome (SIDS)
  - Asthma, chest and ear infections and pneumonia
  - Behaviour problems such as ADHD (attention deficit hyperactivity disorder)
  - Performing poorly at school

both herself and the developing fetus and to correct misinformation. Even if a woman does not choose to make changes due to the information she receives, she still has a right to make an informed choice about her health behaviour.

Activity

Consider the pregnant woman who, when asked by the midwife if she knows the risks of smoking in pregnancy, replies, 'My friend had an 8 lb baby last week and she smoked all the way through her pregnancy'. What would you say to her?

Interventions to help smokers quit

A systematic review concluded that smoking cessation programmes in pregnancy are effective in reducing the number of women who smoke and have a subsequent impact on low birth weight (Chamberlain et al 2017). They identify that there are positive effects of certain forms of counselling, providing feedback and giving incentives to help stop smoking.

NICE (2010b) highlights the role of the midwife in helping women to stop smoking:

1. Identify those who are exposed to tobacco smoke using a carbon monoxide monitor.
2. Identify when the woman last smoked and how many cigarettes she smokes.

3. Provide information about the potential effect of cigarettes on her unborn baby.

4. Explain the health benefits of stopping for the woman and her baby. Advise her to stop, not just cut down.

5. Explain that she will be referred to a specialist midwife or advisor to help her quit.

6. Refer her to NHS Stop Smoking Services and provide the NHS Pregnancy Smoking Helpline number and a local helpline number.

7. Suggest any others in her household who smoke also contact NHS Stop Smoking Services.

8. At the next appointment, check if the woman took up her referral. If not, ask if she is interested in stopping smoking and offer another referral to the service.

The guidance also includes information about following up at subsequent appointments.

Activity

Find out what facilities are available to help pregnant smokers to quit in your locality. Has this service been evaluated? What is the success rate and how is it measured?

Drug dependency

Pregnant drug users have a range of social, emotional and physical needs that require expert attention. This vulnerable group of women requires individualized care. The Confidential Enquiry into Maternal Deaths 2013–15 (Knight et al 2017) identified 17 of the women who died were substance users. Many more women do not die as a result of their drug dependency, but do remain vulnerable because of their chaotic domestic circumstances. The babies of drug users are also at risk of a range of sequelae, depending on the type of drug and degree of abuse (Baston & Durward 2017). NICE (2010c) highlights the fears and anxieties these women may have about the potential of their baby being taken from them and that the attitude of the caregivers is important to maintain their trust.

Women can be referred to local drug dependency services for care and treatment. The benefits of other interventions need further evaluation. Care across the childbirth continuum needs to be carefully coordinated between the members of the multi-professional team. A systematic review to determine the effects of home visits during pregnancy and/or after birth for women with an alcohol or drug problem (Turnbull & Osborn 2012) did not find any health benefits associated with this intervention. There was evidence, however, that home visits after the birth did enhance women's engagement with drug treatment services.

Activity during pregnancy

Fatigue

People often associate fatigue in pregnancy with carrying an extra weight load around. Although this is a factor during the last trimester, it does not explain the debilitating lack of energy in the early weeks. Feeling tired in pregnancy can be extremely frustrating. Early pregnancy is particularly difficult as women have little to show in the way of a swelling abdomen, yet feel that they need to go to bed much earlier than usual. Women need reassurance that it is usual to feel very tired in the first trimester and that it will pass. Partners also need this information as reassurance that they will not spend every evening alone during the pregnancy. Providing feedback regarding the booking full blood count is useful, as women may fear that they are anaemic and this needs to be ruled out or treated.

Activity

What is the midwife looking for when she looks at a full blood count result? Why do some women experience dizziness or fainting when pregnant? What advice can the midwife offer?

Exercise

Moderate exercise during a low-risk pregnancy has not been shown to put the fetus or mother at risk. A recent review for the UK Department of Health (2017) identified that maintaining activity in pregnancy:

1. Reduces hypertensive disorders
2. Improves cardiorespiratory fitness
3. Lowers gestational weight gain
4. Reduces the risk of gestational diabetes

It has the advantage of maintaining flexibility and enhancing self-esteem and has beneficial cardiovascular and respiratory effects. The Royal College of Psychiatrists (2007) recommends exercise to improve mental wellbeing. It has also been identified that diet and exercise interventions reduce the odds of the woman needing a caesarean section (The International Weight Management in Pregnancy (i-WIP) Collaborative Group 2017).

Activity

Access the infographic recommendations on Physical Activity in Pregnancy at

https://www.gov.uk/government/uploads/system/uploads/attachment_data/file/622335/CMO_physical_activity_pregnant_women_infographic.pdf

and the information behind it at https://www.gov.uk/government/uploads/system/uploads/attachment_data/file/622623/Physical_activity_pregnancy_infographic_guidance.pdf

Consider how you may help pregnant women follow this guidance.

Find out what exercise classes are available for pregnant women in your locality.

Contact sports should, however, be avoided, along with those that put excessive stress on the joints, which are more mobile in pregnancy. Women should take measures to avoid over-heating during exercise and ensure that they reduce the risk of hypoglycaemia. Pregnant women should also avoid exercising in the supine position, as this may lead to vena caval compression.

Women who did not previously exercise should be advised to start with non-weightbearing exercise, such as swimming. Regular, moderate exercise is better than sporadic, strenuous exertion, and women should still be able to talk during exercise. Sexual activity during pregnancy for women with an uncomplicated pregnancy is not associated with adverse outcomes (NICE 2008, 2017).

Pelvic girdle pain

Activity may be severely restricted if the woman develops a condition known as *pregnancy-related pelvic girdle pain*. The effect of the hormone relaxin leads to separation of the symphysis pubis, or affects the joints in the pelvis, which in extreme cases makes weightbearing impossible. An estimated one in five women experience this condition (RCOG 2015b). Women who develop this painful condition need a lot of support and individualized care. They should be referred to an obstetric physiotherapist for specialist advice. Treatment is rest, and the condition may persist for several months after the birth or for longer in severe cases.

Backache

Backache affects 50% of pregnant woman (Sabino & Grauer 2008). A combination of increased progesterone and relaxin circulation, increased weight gain and altered posture contributes to pain that can be mild to severe, constant or intermittent. There is evidence that suggests that any form of physical exercise in water or on land will improve backache (Liddle & Pennick 2015). NICE (2008, 2017) suggests that exercise in water, massage and back care classes may help.

Rest during pregnancy

Although moderate exercise is beneficial during pregnancy, a balance between activity and rest that meets the individual woman's requirement is optimum. There is no evidence that rest should be enforced on women, for example, to reduce the risk of preterm birth (Sosa et al 2015). Unfortunately, many women experience difficulties maintaining their pre-pregnancy sleeping patterns, and this can be a source of anxiety. Pregnant women may experience disturbed sleep patterns for many reasons, and this may be a sign of depressive conditions (Paavonen et al 2017). The midwife needs to carefully explore a range of issues with women who complain of lack of or disturbed sleep to give appropriate advice. Ultimately, the woman may need to alter her usual sleep and rest patterns during her pregnancy.

Uncomfortable in bed

Women who had previously slept on their front may soon find that this position is no longer possible due to an enlarging abdomen and/or breast tenderness. It can be helpful not only to suggest but also to demonstrate how a pillow under the abdomen and one in between the legs can help a woman sleep comfortably on her side. It is not advisable for pregnant women to sleep on their back, as the weight of the gravid uterus on the vena cava can impede venous return, causing a drop in blood pressure and oxygen supply to the fetus. Women are also more likely to snore in pregnancy, due to changes in nasal mucosa, and this may be worse for those with high BMI at the start of pregnancy and oedema (Sarberg et al 2014).

Sleep position

There is growing evidence based on research in New Zealand that going to sleep on her back increases a woman's chances of having a stillbirth by 3.7 times (McCowan et al 2017). This may be a consequence of reduced pressure on the vena cava and reduced blood flow through the uterine artery in this position. Further research in the UK (Heazell et al 2018) showed a 2.3 time risk of stillbirth if a woman fell asleep on her back. A public health campaign is now underway to 'Sleep on Side' (https://www.tommys.org/pregnancy-information/sleep-side/sleep-side-late-pregnancy-campaign-film).

Fetal movements at night

Women tend to notice the baby's movements more during a rest period because their work or general activities do not distract them. Also, the baby seems to enjoy the increased blood flow and oxygen supply, as they are not competing with active muscles. Fetal movements are a sign of wellbeing and should be enjoyed; however, the woman may need help to relax in spite of her active baby. Simple relaxation techniques can be practised, and a warm bath before bedtime may help as the baby can have its active period then, instead of when the woman gets into bed.

Cramp

Cramp of the legs can be severe, bringing an abrupt end to a deep sleep. Exercising the muscles before bedtime by rapid and repeated flexion and extension of each foot can help disperse the buildup of lactic acid that causes the pain. During an acute attack of cramp, the offending foot should be pulled towards the body to extend the calf muscle (easier said than done when heavily pregnant). Alternatively, the foot can be pressed against the wall or the woman can stand up with the leg behind the body (but this involves getting out of bed). A systematic review of interventions for leg cramps in pregnancy concluded that there is current limited evidence to suggest any medications will help with relief of these symptoms (Zhou et al 2015).

Aching legs

Progesterone relaxes vascular tone, making the valves in the veins less effective and impeding venous return. Compounded by the pressure exerted by the gravid uterus, development of varicose veins in the legs and perineal region can be problematic. In addition, uncomfortable, fidgety legs are often an irritation during pregnancy. Gentle exercise, such as ankle rotation, can provide temporary relief. The woman can be advised to elevate her legs while sitting, if possible. Support tights may also help and prevent or reduce oedema.

Frequency of micturition

This is a problem particularly in the first and third trimesters of pregnancy. In the first trimester the growing uterus is a pelvic organ and shares the space with the bladder. Women need to be reassured that this problem will pass (albeit to return later), and it is useful to show a picture demonstrating the position of the pelvic and abdominal contents in relation to one another to help her appreciate how her body is changing. In the last few weeks of pregnancy, as the presenting part enters the pelvis, there is the same competition for space. However, there is the additional factor that the baby can move its head or bottom and exert pressure on the already compromised bladder, resulting in an urgent need for the woman to pass urine. In addition, her kidneys will be increasing output due to the need to remove more waste from her body. It is recommended that the woman continue to drink fluids, cutting down on caffeine, as this may be an irritant to the bladder, and potentially reducing the amount she drinks before going to bed. However, night waking is likely to remain. There also needs to be awareness of the potential for urinary tract infection and careful questioning to exclude this.

Activity

Find out how a woman's bowel may be affected by pregnancy. What advice is given to women with constipation in pregnancy?

Carpal tunnel syndrome

This condition is not exclusive to pregnancy, but can arise during pregnancy in women who have not experienced it at other times. It is caused by swelling or compression in the space in the wrist where the nerve travels to the hand. It results in pain and/or paresthesia in the hand, which then leads the woman to wake up. Diagnosis of the condition is not easy, and developments using electrodiagnosis are being investigated (Basiri & Katirji 2015). The woman may not realize at first what is waking her up. Elevating the arm on a pillow or the use of a splint may provide some relief, but the condition may not resolve until after the birth.

Activity

Is oedema normal during pregnancy? How and when should the midwife assess the woman for the development of varicose veins? Why do varicose veins need to be observed? What advice can the midwife offer? What treatment is recommended in your locality?

REFLECTION ON THE TRIGGER SCENARIO

Look back on the trigger scenario.

Joanna is now 20 weeks pregnant. She has been well, although rather nauseous at times, but this is now less frequent. She gave up smoking 3 weeks ago and is now beginning to struggle. She even got to the stage where she took one of Louis's cigarettes from the packet and searched through the kitchen drawer to find a lighter that worked. She was interrupted by an interesting text message and then managed to gather her willpower to put the cigarette back in its packet.

The scenario highlights how addressing a health behaviour, such as smoking, can be challenging and difficult to achieve alone. It also emphasizes the need to engage women's partners in the experience of pregnancy, as well as recognize the social context of the woman, so that they can provide support and prepare for their new role. Now that you are familiar with the issues in relation to health in pregnancy, you should have insight into how the scenario relates to the evidence. The jigsaw model will now be used to explore the trigger scenario in more depth.

Effective communication

Joanna has decided to give up smoking, and this is going well so far. However, she has found that she is filling the time she would usually be spending smoking with eating, and this has led to a significant weight gain in a relatively short period.

Questions that arise from the scenario might include the following: How has Joanna received the message that she should give up smoking during pregnancy? Has it come from a health professional or through the media, family or peer group? What is the most effective method of changing health behaviours? How are women encouraged to access information about healthy lifestyles where you work?

Woman-centred care

Information about health in pregnancy should be specific to the individual needs of the woman. Questions that arise from the scenario might include the following: Did Joanna receive tailored information about her smoking habit at the booking history? Was the information given relevant and applicable to her current circumstances? Were her questions answered and any need for referral followed up? Was Joanna given information about local services that could help her address her smoking habit? Was an individual plan developed and documented with a plan for review discussed? How was Louis included in Joanna's plans to quit smoking?

Using best evidence

Many interventions are available to help women stop smoking, some specifically for those who are pregnant. Questions that arise from the scenario might include the following: Were different options for support to stop smoking discussed with Joanna? How are midwives informed of the most effective methods available? Are there evidence-based programmes of care available in your locality? Is there an evidence-based policy or pathway available for use when a pregnant woman books for maternity care? Do you know how many pregnant smokers attempt to stop smoking and succeed? Is there an on-going audit of local smoking cessation programmes? What do the NICE guidelines recommend about smoking in pregnancy?

Professional and legal issues

It is part of the midwife's role to offer advice in pregnancy and to counsel women about their health behaviours (ICM 2017). Questions that arise from the scenario might include the following: How do midwives keep up to date with new evidence about health in pregnancy? Are workshops/information sessions provided at the trust where you work? How can you identify and address your learning needs? What might be the potential consequences if you did not inform a woman about the risks she was taking by continuing to smoke during pregnancy? How do you document the advice you have given to women?

Team working

The midwife works as part of a team of professionals, each with an area of expertise and experience. Questions that arise from the scenario might include the following: Which professionals will Joanna already have come into contact with by this stage of her pregnancy? Which professionals would be best placed to discuss smoking cessation? Is there someone in your locality with a specific role in supporting pregnant women to stop smoking? What do you do when an issue is outside your level of expertise? How do you communicate with other members of the healthcare team?

Clinical dexterity

The midwife who refers a woman for help with smoking cessation will need an understanding of the techniques that are used to support this process even if she does not use them herself. The most important clinical skill will be sensitive interview techniques to gather accurate information and provide genuine emotional support. In addition she must be able to use a carbon monoxide monitor and interpret the results. Questions that arise from the scenario might include the following: What interventions are used in your locality to support pregnant women who smoke? What do nicotine patches look like and how are they applied? How much nicotine do the patches prescribed in pregnancy contain? Are patches worn all day? What other nicotine replacement products are available?

Models of care

The model of care that the woman is following could have significant implications for her success in making a change to her smoking status.

This applies not only to the model of maternity care (e.g. is she receiving continuous support from a midwife?) but also with regard to the smoking cessation programme she is following. Questions that arise from the scenario might include the following: Does the antenatal documentation enable all professionals involved in care to follow Joanna's progress? Is Joanna supported on a one-to-one basis or is there a local group for peer support? Are processes in place to enable Joanna to seek advice and support in between appointments?

Safe environment

The midwife needs to ensure that she provides a safe environment for women to disclose their individual circumstances so that appropriate individualized care can be offered. She also needs to monitor that pre-scribed treatments or interventions are being used appropriately. Questions that arise from the scenario might include the following: Is there sufficient privacy and time within the provision of antenatal care to enable women to disclose their concerns? How can the current system/environment be adapted to enhance communication? What is the regime for smoking cessation intervention locally?

Promotes health

The midwife has many opportunities throughout the antenatal period to promote the current and future health of women and their families. Questions that arise from the scenario might include the following: If Joanna quits smoking in pregnancy, how can she be supported to continue her abstinence once the baby is born? How can the midwife use this opportunity to promote the health of the baby? What information can the midwife give Joanna that will help her confront members of the family who smoke and prepare them to maintain a smoke-free environment for the new baby?

Further scenarios

The following scenarios enable you to consider how specific situations influence the care the midwife provides. Use the jigsaw model to explore the issues raised in the scenario.

SCENARIO 1

Lisa has given up smoking but she has become rather fond of the pastries on sale at the shop near her work. She is 22 weeks pregnant and has already put on over 6 kg in weight.

Practice point

It has been highlighted previously that women do not need extra calories for pregnancy until the final trimester. In usual circumstances the most weight gain will also take place in the later stages of pregnancy. Increased weight gain at such an early stage is therefore something to take note of.

Further questions specific to Scenario 1 include:

1. How many extra calories does Lisa need?
2. What strategies can the midwife suggest to help Lisa from putting on unnecessary weight?
3. How can Lisa safely increase her physical activity in pregnancy?
4. NICE guidance states that repeated weighing during pregnancy should only be undertaken if it might influence clinical management (NICE 2008, 2017). How might this be interpreted?
5. Which other members of the healthcare team could potentially support Lisa to eat a balanced diet?

SCENARIO 2

Lucy has just found out she is 6 weeks pregnant. She is a keen horse rider about to take part in a national competition and contacts her local community midwife for advice about continuing with this sport.

Practice point

Understanding of activity and sport has evolved in recent years with recognition for those who are already aware of fitness in comparison to those who do not undertake regular activity. Complications arise with sports such as horse riding, where some potential danger is involved. The decision to continue may therefore be related to the understanding of risk for the woman herself. It is also to be remembered that despite advice that may be given, it remains the woman's choice whether she continues.

Further questions specific to Scenario 2 include:

1. What does the evidence say about horse riding in pregnancy?
2. What other sources of information are available to women?
3. What are the potential risks and benefits of Lucy continuing to ride while pregnant?
4. What are your own personal feelings about competitive sports and pregnancy?
5. What is your role as a midwife in relation to giving advice?

Conclusion

Pregnancy makes many emotional and physical demands on the woman. She will value the support and experience of the midwives who care for her as she faces new challenges and makes choices about her lifestyle. The midwife has an important public health role that reaches beyond the childbirth continuum.

Resources

Bump It Up: The Dynamic, Flexible Exercise and Healthy Eating Plan For Before, During and After Pregnancy 2016 Author: Greg Whyte, Penguin Books

Read more at https://www.penguin.co.uk/books/1111959/bump-it-up/#G6FssrOXk3quB9wg.99

Department of Health

http://www.dh.gov.uk/en/index.htm

Healthy Start

http://www.healthystart.nhs.uk/

Pelvic Obstetric and Gynaecological Physiotherapy

http://pogp.csp.org.uk/about-pogp

Pregnancy Sickness Support

https://www.pregnancysicknesssupport.org.uk/help/women-suffering/hyperemesis-gravidarum/

Stop Smoking

http://www.nhs.uk/livewell/smoking/Pages/stopsmokingnewhome.aspx

Side to Sleep campaign

https://www.tommys.org/pregnancy-information/sleep-side/sleep-side-late-pregnancy-campaign-film

References

Basiri, K., Katirji, B., 2015. Practical approach to electrodiagnosis of the carpal tunnel syndrome: a review. Adv. Biomed. Res. 4, 50. doi:10.4103/2277-9175.151552. eCollection 2015.

Baston, H., Durward, H., 2017. Examination of the Newborn, third ed. Routledge, London.

Bayol, S.A., Simbi, B.H., Bertrand, J.A., Stickland, N.C., 2008. Offspring from mothers fed a "junk food" diet in pregnancy and lactation exhibit exacerbated adiposity that is more pronounced in females. J. Physiol. 586 (Pt 13), 3219–3230. doi:10.1113/jphysiol.2008.153817.

Care study group, 2008. Maternal caffeine intake during pregnancy and risk of fetal growth restriction: a large prospective observational study. BMJ 337, a2332.

Chamberlain, C., O'Mara-Eves, A., Porter, J., et al., 2017. Psychosocial interventions for supporting women to stop smoking in pregnancy. Cochrane Database Syst. Rev. (2), Art. No.: CD001055, doi:10.1002/14651858.CD001055.pub5.

Chen, L., Yi Wu, N., Foong-Fong Chong, M., et al., 2014. Maternal caffeine intake during pregnancy is associated with risk of low birth weight: a systematic review and dose–response meta-analysis. BMC Med. 12 (1), 174. doi:10.1186/s12916-014-0174-6. Http://dx.doi.org/10.1186/s12916-014-0174-6. Web.

Claesson, I., Sydsjo, G., Brynhildsen, J., et al., 2008. Weight gain restriction for obese pregnant women: a case control intervention study. BJOG 115 (1), 44–50.

Coad, J., Dunstall, M., 2011. Anatomy and Physiology for Midwives, third ed. Elsevier Health sciences, Oxford.

Department of Health, 2016. UK Chief Medical Officers' Alcohol Guidelines Review. http://www.drugsandalcohol.ie/25010/1/CMO_UK_Alcohol_guidelines _review_summary.pdf.

Department of Health, 2017. Physical activity in pregnancy infographic: guidance. https://www.gov.uk/government/uploads/system/uploads/attachment_data/ file/622623/Physical_activity_pregnancy_infographic_guidance.pdf.

Duley, L., Henderson-Smart, D., Meher, S., 2005. Altered dietary salt for preventing pre-eclampsia, and its complications. Cochrane Database Syst. Rev. (4), CD005548.

First Steps Nutrition Trust, 2017. Eating well for a healthy pregnancy: a practical guide. http://www.firststepsnutrition.org/pdfs/Eating_Well_for_a_healthy _Pregnancy_2017.pdf.

Grieger, J.A., Clifton, V.L., 2015. A review of the impact of dietary intakes in human pregnancy on infant birthweight. Nutrients 7 (1), 153–178. doi:10.3390/ nu7010153.

Heazell, A.E.P., Li, M., Budd, J., et al., 2018. Association between maternal sleep practices and late stillbirth – findings from a stillbirth case-control study. BJOG 125, 254–262.

Institute of Medicine, 2009. Weight Gain During Pregnancy: Reexamining the Guidelines. http://www.nationalacademies.org/hmd/~/media/Files/Report%20 Files/2009/Weight-Gain-During-Pregnancy-Reexamining-the-Guidelines/ Report%20Brief%20-%20Weight%20Gain%20During%20Pregnancy.pdf.

International Confederation of Midwives (ICM), 2017. International Definition of the Midwife. Available from: http://internationalmidwives.org/assets/uploads/ documents/CoreDocuments/ENG%20Definition_of_the_Midwife%202017.pdf.

Janakiraman, V., 2008. Listeriosis in pregnancy: diagnosis, treatment, and prevention. Rev. Obstet. Gynecol. 1 (4), 179–185.

Jewell, K., 2017. Nutrition. In: MacDonald, S., Johnson, G. (Eds.), Mayes Midwifery. Elsevier, London.

Klebanoff, M.A., Harper, M., Lai, Y., et al., 2011. Fish consumption, erythrocyte fatty acids, and preterm birth. Obstet. Gynecol. 117 (5), 1071–1077. http:// doi.org/10.1097/AOG.0b013e31821645dc.

Knight, M., Nair, M., Tuffnell, D., et al., (Eds.) on behalf of MBRRACE-UK, 2017. Saving Lives, Improving Mothers' Care - Lessons learned to inform maternity care from the UK and Ireland Confidential Enquiries into Maternal Deaths and Morbidity 2013–15. National Perinatal Epidemiology Unit, University of Oxford, Oxford. https://www.npeu.ox.ac.uk/downloads/files/mbrrace-uk/ reports/MBRRACE-UK%20Maternal%20Report%202017%20-%20Web.pdf.

Liddle, S.D., Pennick, V., 2015. Interventions for preventing and treating low-back and pelvic pain during pregnancy. Cochrane Database Syst. Rev. (9), Art. No.: CD001139, doi:10.1002/14651858.CD001139.pub4.

McCarthy, F.P., Lutomski, J.E., Greene, R.A., 2014. Hyperemesis gravidarum: current perspectives. Int. J. Womens Health 6, 719–725. http://doi.org/10.2147/ IJWH.S37685.

McCowan, L., John, M., Thompson, R., et al., 2017. Going to sleep in the supine position is a modifiable risk factor for late pregnancy stillbirth; findings from the New Zealand multicentre stillbirth case-control study. PLoS ONE 12 (6), e0179396.

NICE, 2008, 2014. Maternal and child nutrition. https://www.nice.org.uk/guidance/ph11/chapter/2-Public-health-need-and-practice#socioeconomic-influences-on-maternal-and-child-nutrition.

NICE, 2008, 2017. Antenatal care for uncomplicated pregnancies clinical guideline. https://www.nice.org.uk/guidance/cg62.

NICE, 2010a. Weight management before, during and after pregnancy. https://www.nice.org.uk/guidance/ph27/chapter/1-Recommendations#recommendation-2-pregnant-women.

NICE, 2010b. Smoking: stopping in pregnancy and after childbirth. https://www.nice.org.uk/guidance/ph26/chapter/1-Recommendations#effective-interventions.

NICE, 2010c. Pregnancy and complex social factors: a model for service provision for pregnant women with complex social factors. https://www.nice.org.uk/guidance/CG110/chapter/1-Guidance#pregnant-women-who-misuse-substances-alcohol-andor-drugs.

NICE, 2011. Hypertension in pregnancy: diagnosis and management. https://www.nice.org.uk/guidance/cg107/chapter/1-Guidance#management-of-pregnancy-with-chronic-hypertension.

Olsen, S.F., Secher, N.J., 2002. Low consumption of seafood in early pregnancy as a factor for preterm delivery: a prospective cohort study. Br. Med. J. 324 (7335), 447–450.

Ota, E., Hori, H., Mori, R., et al., 2015. Antenatal dietary education and supplementation to increase energy and protein intake. Cochrane Database Syst. Rev. (6), Art. No.: CD000032, doi:10.1002/14651858.CD000032.pub3.

Ovesen, P., Tasmussen, S., Kesmodel, U., 2011. Effect of prepregnancy maternal overweight and obesity on pregnancy outcome. Obstetrics & Gynecology 118 (2 Pt 1), 305–312.

Paavonen, J., Saarenpää-Heikkilä, O., Pölkki, P., et al., 2017. Maternal and paternal sleep during pregnancy in the Child-Sleep birth cohort. Sleep Med. 29, 47–56. doi:10.1016/j.sleep.2016.09.011. [Epub 2016 Nov 4].

Peña-Rosas, J.P., De-Regil, L.M., Garcia-Casal, M.N., Dowswell, T., 2015. Daily oral iron supplementation during pregnancy. Cochrane Database Syst. Rev. (7), Art. No.: CD004736, doi:10.1002/14651858.CD004736.pub5.

Platts, J., Mitchell, E., Stacey, T., et al., 2014. The Midland and North of England Stillbirth Study (MiNESS). BMC Pregnancy Childbirth 14, 171. Web.

Public Health England, 2016. The Eatwell Guide. Available from: http://www.nhs.uk/Livewell/Goodfood/Documents/The-Eatwell-Guide-2016.pdf.

Rankin, J., Tennant, P.W.G., Stothard, K.J., et al., 2010. Maternal body mass index and congenital anomaly risk: a cohort study. Int. J. Obes. 34 (9), 1371–1380.

Rhee, J., Kim, R., Kim, Y., et al., 2015. Maternal Caffeine Consumption during Pregnancy and Risk of Low Birth Weight: A Dose-Response Meta-Analysis of Observational Studies. PLoS ONE 10 (7), e0132334. http://doi.org/10.1371/journal.pone.0132334.

Richens, Y., 2008. Tackling maternal obesity: suggestions for midwives. Br. J. Midwifery 16 (1), 14–18.

RCOG, 2006. Alcohol consumption and the outcomes of pregnancy. Statement No 5 http://www.alcoholpolicy.net/files/RCOG_Alcohol_pregnancy_March_06.pdf.

RCOG, 2015a. Smoking and pregnancy. https://www.rcog.org.uk/globalassets/documents/patients/patient-information-leaflets/pregnancy/pi-smoking-and-pregnancy-2.pdf.

RCOG, 2015b. Pelvic girdle pain and pregnancy. https://www.rcog.org.uk/globalassets/documents/patients/patient-information-leaflets/pregnancy/pi-pelvic-girdle-pain-and-pregnancy.pdf.

Royal College of Psychiatrists, 2007. Mental Health in Pregnancy. http://www.rcpsych.ac.uk/expertadvice/problems/mentalhealthinpregnancy.aspx.

Rungsiprakarn, P., Laopaiboon, M., Sangkomkamhang, U.S., et al., 2015. Interventions for treating constipation in pregnancy. Cochrane Database Syst. Rev. (9), Art. No.: CD011448, doi:10.1002/14651858.CD011448.pub2.

Sabino, J., Grauer, J.N., 2008. Pregnancy and low back pain. Curr. Rev. Musculoskelet. Med. 1 (2), 137–141. http://doi.org/10.1007/s12178-008-9021-8.

Sarberg, M., Svanborg, E., Wiréhn, A.B., Josefsson, A., 2014. Snoring during pregnancy and its relation to sleepiness and pregnancy outcome - a prospective study. BMC Pregnancy Childbirth 14, 15. doi:10.1186/1471-2393-14-15.

Shalini, O., Fainberg, P., Sebert, S., et al., 2015. Maternal health and eating habits: metabolic consequences and impact on child health. Trends Mol. Med. 21 (2), 126–133. Web.

Sosa, C.G., Althabe, F., Belizán, J.M., Bergel, E., 2015. Bed rest in singleton pregnancies for preventing preterm birth. Cochrane Database Syst. Rev. (3), CD003581, doi:10.1002/14651858.CD003581.pub3.

Thaxter Nesbeth, K.A., Samuels, L.A., Nicholson, D.C., et al., 2016. Ptyalism in pregnancy – a review of epidemiology and practices. Eur. J. Obstet. Gynecol. Reprod. Biol. 198, 47–49.

The International Weight Management in Pregnancy (i-WIP) Collaborative Group, 2017. Effect of diet and physical activity based interventions in pregnancy on gestational weight gain and pregnancy outcomes: meta-analysis of individual participant data from randomised trials. BMJ 358, j3119, doi:10.1136/bmj.j3119.

Tieu, J., Shepherd, E., Middleton, P., Crowther, C.A., 2017. Dietary advice interventions in pregnancy for preventing gestational diabetes mellitus. Cochrane Database Syst. Rev. (1), Art. No.: CD006674, doi:10.1002/14651858.CD006674.pub3.

Turnbull, C., Osborn, D.A., 2012. Home visits during pregnancy and after birth for women with an alcohol or drug problem. Cochrane Database Syst. Rev. (1), CD004456, doi:10.1002/14651858.CD004456.pub3.

Wald, N., Sneddon, J., Densem, J., et al., 1991. Prevention of neural tube defects: results of the medical research council vitamin study. Lancet 338 (8760), 131–137.

Zhou, K., West, H.M., Zhang, J., et al., 2015. Interventions for leg cramps in pregnancy. Cochrane Database Syst. Rev. (8), CD010655, doi:10.1002/14651858.CD010655.pub2.

CHAPTER 5

Monitoring maternal physical wellbeing

TRIGGER SCENARIO

Joanna is now 25 weeks pregnant. She has just returned from her antenatal checkup with the midwife. It was not the same midwife who had taken her booking history, but she was friendly and took time to read through Jo's records. The midwife said that her blood pressure was up a bit, but when she retook it later it was fine. Jo had meant to ask her midwife what she should take for heartburn, but did not get the chance. She will call in at the chemist on her way to work.

Introduction

This chapter focuses on aspects of the 'antenatal check' undertaken by the midwife that monitor the physical wellbeing of the pregnant woman. Previous chapters have examined the procedure and rationale for some of the clinical activities undertaken by the midwife to assess the woman's health status. During assessment of maternal physical health, the midwife will undertake an evaluation of her emotional wellbeing, and issues surrounding this aspect of care will be considered in further detail in the following chapter. Aspects of the examination that address assessment of fetal wellbeing, including abdominal palpation, will be discussed in Chapter 9.

The antenatal check

The National Institute for Health and Care Excellence (NICE) has published recommendations regarding the content and frequency of antenatal appointments (NICE 2008, 2017) and these are summarized in Table 5.1. It is recommended that, after their initial contact with a health professional to confirm pregnancy, nulliparous women should have 10 antenatal appointments and multiparous women should have 7 (NICE 2008, 2017).

A large national survey of women's experience of maternity care (Redshaw & Henderson 2015) reported that there was little difference between the mean number of antenatal checks for women who had babies

Table 5.1: Schedule of antenatal contacts and their content

When	Primparous	Multiparous
First contact with a health professional: confirmation of pregnancy.		
Booking (by 10 weeks)	Blood tests for blood group, rhesus factor, anaemia, haemoglobinopathies, red cell alloantibodies, hepatitis B virus, HIV and syphilis. Offer dating and anomaly scans and information on antenatal screening tests, healthy eating and vitamin D supplementation. Calculate Body Mass Index (BMI), blood pressure (BP), test urine for protein, MSU for asymptomatic bacteriuria. Carbon monoxide (CO) monitoring and referral to stop smoking service for all women who smoke.	
10–14 weeks	If chosen, ultrasound scan to determine gestational age and Down's syndrome screening from 11–13 weeks 6 days (combined test) or 15–20 weeks (triple or quadruple). If mother is rhesus D-negative, some maternity units offer a blood test to identify the rhesus D status of the fetus and cell-free fetal DNA (cffDNA) so that routine antenatal anti-D prophylaxis (RAADP), can be avoided if fetus is rhesus D negative. CO monitoring.	
16 weeks	BP, urinalysis and CO monitoring. Review screening tests, information giving.	
18–20 weeks	If chosen, structural anomaly scan, placental localization	
25 weeks	BP, urinalysis and CO monitoring. Information giving, measurement and plotting of symphysis–fundal height, Inquire about fetal activity, MAT B1 form provided.	No routine visit
28 weeks	BP, urinalysis and CO monitoring. Information giving, measurement and plotting of symphysis–fundal height, offer anti-D prophylaxis to rhesus-negative women (where the fetal rhesus D status is unknown (cffDNA not performed) or the fetus is known to be rhesus D positive). Screen for anaemia and atypical red cell alloantibodies, inquire about fetal activity.	
31 weeks	BP, urinalysis and CO monitoring. Information giving, measurement and plotting of symphysis–fundal height. Inquire about fetal activity. Review blood screening.	No routine visit
34 weeks	BP, urinalysis and CO monitoring. Information giving, measurement and plotting of symphysis–fundal height (offer second anti-D prophylaxis to rhesus-negative women – some maternity units only). Inquire about fetal activity.	

Continued

Table 5.1: Schedule of antenatal contacts and their content (Continued)

When	Primparous	Multiparous
36 weeks	BP, urinalysis and CO monitoring. Information giving – preparation for birth, postnatal awareness, measurement and plotting of symphysis–fundal height. Check position and presentation of baby. Inquire about fetal activity.	
38 weeks	BP, urinalysis and CO monitoring. Measurement and plotting of symphysis–fundal height, information giving, inquire about fetal activity.	
40 weeks	BP, urinalysis and CO monitoring. Measurement and plotting of symphysis–fundal height. Information giving, inquire about fetal activity.	No routine visit
41 weeks	BP, urinalysis and CO monitoring. Information giving, measurement and plotting of symphysis–fundal height. Offer a membrane sweep. Offer induction of labour. Inquire about fetal activity.	

before (10.1 vs. 9.5), with an overall average of 10 checks. After review of the evidence, the World Health Organization (WHO) has revised its recommendations from four focused visits to a minimum of eight antenatal contacts (WHO 2016).

Women in all settings are less satisfied with fewer visits, and some feel that the gap between visits is too long (Dowswell et al 2015).

Table 5.1 shows a schedule of antenatal appointments for primiparous and multiparous women, together with the content of the visits. See Chapter 7 for more information about blood tests in pregnancy.

The midwife should be mindful that the NICE antenatal care guideline is aimed at 'healthy pregnant women' and where women need more support or additional monitoring, this should be scheduled accordingly. Ultimately care should be tailored to meet the needs of individual women and a personalized care plan developed with her (The National Maternity Review 2016). For example, a woman experiencing a normal second pregnancy may not need to be seen as often as a woman who has a history of infertility. However, this assumption is based on generalization. The woman expecting her second baby may have had a traumatic first birth or a sister who has had a stillbirth. She may require a lot of additional support from the professionals she meets. The woman with a history of infertility may be happy and well and content to be seen according to the usual schedule. Where possible, continuity of carer should be aimed for (The National Maternity Review 2016); one of the many benefits of continuity of antenatal care is that the midwife can establish and maintain relationships with women, noticing when circumstances change and when the way care is offered needs to adapt in response.

Record keeping

Throughout midwifery practice, our records facilitate effective care and can be used to repeat and confirm our assessment and plan of action with the woman. She should be shown what is written so that it can be explained there and then, rather than her going away and wondering what it all means. At the end of the interaction, the woman should understand the implications of any findings and what happens next. Finally, she should be invited to ask any more questions. Many maternity units are using electronic care records and giving women access to these through bespoke apps or websites. Following the National Maternity Review (2016), NHS Digital is working with maternity units with the ultimate aim of women having access to records that are interoperable. This will enable women to both read and contribute to their own records and access evidence-based information to inform their decisions.

Safety

The woman attending her antenatal checkup has probably been anticipating it (either with joy or dread) for several days beforehand. She may have thought of questions she wanted to ask or have been worried that her blood pressure might be up again. Women want to work in partnership with their healthcare professionals (The National Maternity Review 2016). In a study by Boyle et al (2016), a partnership relationship was defined as:

> *A dynamic relationship that recognises the autonomy of both partners and is based on mutual co-operation and shared responsibility. It enables reciprocity and facilitates shared decision making through a process of negotiation based on trust and respect, recognising and valuing the experiences that each partner brings to the relationship.*
>
> (Boyle et al 2016:24)

The challenge for the midwife with many women to see in a busy antenatal clinic is to enable each woman to feel that she has been treated with respect and as an individual. Staff shortages, study leave and sickness compound to make this a tall order. However, eye contact, acknowledgement and active listening will enhance the interaction without substantially lengthening the consultation. When a woman obviously needs more time, depending on the structure of local services and her current health status, it may be possible to offer a home visit or schedule another appointment.

The woman must feel that the room is safe, that the door will not suddenly be opened and a private conversation or disclosure interrupted. She also needs to feel that the information she offers will not be passed around the staff room or to the next woman in the waiting room. She will judge this by the midwife's interactions with her. For example, if the midwife is not telling her about the previous person or the woman who lives next door, then this will give her more confidence that the midwife will not discuss her circumstances with others either.

Emotional wellbeing

The emotions that women experience during their pregnancy are wide ranging. They may change over the duration of the pregnancy and differ between individual pregnancies. The woman may need to explore her feelings with a midwife, and an opening question such as 'How are you feeling?' provides such an opportunity.

The mind and body are inextricably linked such that physical pathology may lead to emotional distress and vice versa. The midwife also needs to recognize the impact of maternal ill health on the wellbeing of the developing baby and, conversely, that concern about the baby will affect the emotional health of the woman. The woman's general activity level and sprightliness may speak volumes, not just about her physical health, but also regarding her emotional health. In clinic situations, it is good practice to go out to the waiting room and call the woman in personally. Doing so enables the midwife to assess her mobility and her mood. We can all put on a smile, but much more than that is difficult to maintain if we are feeling low. Our body gives us away by our posture and eye contact. See Chapter 6 for further insights into monitoring a woman's emotional wellbeing in pregnancy.

Activity

Identify an example of how the discovery of physical illness in the mother could lead to her emotional distress. How would you minimize its effect? Find out what services are available in your locality for pregnant women with mental health problems.

Social activity

Showing interest in the woman, rather than just the progress of the pregnancy, demonstrates concern for her as an individual. Knowledge of what the woman is doing will also provide insight into how she is feeling. It would be inappropriate to bombard the woman with a list of probing questions, but the midwife will need to satisfy herself that she is aware of the woman's social circumstances, particularly if she did not do the booking history at the woman's home. Is she getting support from her partner and are they making preparations together? Does she have family and friends in the area, or is the woman socially isolated?

It is also important to follow up on issues that were highlighted during the booking history. For example, if the woman smoked and showed an interest in quitting, it is important to find out how her plans are going. She may have initially declined referral to a local support initiative, but now feels that she would like to take up the offer. If she has stopped smoking, continued support, praise and encouragement may help her maintain her resolve.

Physical tests
Routine urinalysis

It is recommended that the woman's urine is tested for proteinuria at each antenatal examination (NICE 2008, 2017). She is asked to provide a midstream specimen in a clean container. Although a washed-out jar or bottle will suffice, a specimen bottle is more discrete and secure and can be washed and reused throughout the pregnancy. Proteinuria is an ominous symptom of pre-eclampsia. There should not be any protein in urine; however, detection of a trace of protein may be present through contamination and does not require further action unless associated with other signs of pathology.

Activity

Think about how you might discuss the finding of proteinuria with a woman. Work out how you might explain the significance without alarming her. Make sure you know what further tests or follow-up might be indicated.

Blood pressure measurement

Due to the successful implementation of evidence practice in relation to hypertensive disease in pregnancy, it kills 1 woman every 18 months compared with 150 women 60 years ago (Harding et al 2016). Vigilance is paramount, and blood pressure should be measured and recorded at each antenatal examination (NICE 2008, 2017). Women whose blood pressure falls outside the normal range: x2 reading of >90 mm Hg more than 4 hours apart and/or +1 of protein, or x1 reading of 110 mm Hg, should be reviewed (NICE 2008, 2017). This may involve referral to an antenatal day assessment unit where her blood pressure can be monitored over time, with urine and blood analysis as per NICE guidance (2010a, 2011).

Depending on the circumstances and local policy, the woman may be referred to an antenatal assessment unit for further monitoring. In the absence of proteinurea, other symptoms and a relatively small increase from the booking blood pressure reading, the midwife may arrange to repeat the blood pressure measurement in the woman's own home. Women should be informed to contact the hospital if they experience visual disturbances, severe headache or epigastric pain. However, many women with pre-eclampsia feel well. For detailed instruction on how to take an accurate blood pressure, see *Midwifery Essentials: Basics* (Baston & Hall 2017).

Activity

Find out about Korotkoff sounds. Make sure you know which you should record during pregnancy.

Think of five questions you might ask the woman if her blood pressure is raised.

Carbon monoxide (CO) screening

Carbon monoxide is a colourless, odourless, poisonous gas that is produced through combustion. It combines readily with haemoglobin and thus reduces the oxygen-carrying capacity of the blood, thereby reducing the oxygen supply to the developing fetus. It is recommended that all pregnant women are offered CO screening at each antenatal contact (NICE 2010b, 2013) and that women with CO levels of 4 ppm are asked about the potential source of exposure (National Centre for Smoking Cessation and Training (NCSCT 2014)). CO is found in cigarette smoke and vehicle exhaust emissions and can also be produced from faulty gas appliances and wood-burning stoves. Women who smoke or who have recently quit should be referred to a stop smoking service for behavioural and/or pharmacological support.

Blood tests

The booking blood results should be available and documented in the woman's maternity records by the 16-week appointment (NICE 2008, 2017). The woman should be informed of all results and their meaning should be explained. Abnormal results should be discussed with the woman and a clear plan of action documented. See Chapter 7 for further details regarding blood tests in pregnancy.

Clinical examination and inquiry

Legs

Thromboembolism is the leading *direct* (related to pregnancy or childbirth) cause of maternal death in the United Kingdom (Knight et al 2016). The midwife should ask the woman if she has any pain in her legs and assess them by looking to see that they are both the same size (different sizes might occur if there is a deep vein thrombosis in the calf – measure them if there is any uncertainty). Uncomfortable varicose veins might benefit from support tights, but need careful monitoring for the development of phlebitis.

Tight, shiny skin may be present if the woman has marked oedema. If present, the midwife assesses the severity by asking how far up the leg it goes and gently depressing the skin in front of the tibia, to see if the skin remains depressed when the finger is removed. The farther up the leg the indentation can be made, the more severe the oedema. The midwife should also ask if the oedema goes down at night, which it should. The hands and face should also be assessed. Although oedema is both common and normal in pregnancy, it can be associated with pre-eclampsia and should alert the midwife to exclude the development of this condition. Also, common or not, it is still uncomfortable and does not enhance the body image. The midwife can offer simple advice regarding elevating legs when seated and regular leg exercises to improve venous return, but most importantly she should provide reassurance and understanding.

Vaginal loss

Any report of vaginal loss of fluid needs careful investigation. Bleeding in pregnancy is abnormal and necessitates further investigation to identify the cause. Women need to know the difference between a 'show' and antepartum haemorrhage. A 'show' is always mixed with mucus. Blood that soaks through the pants or runs down the leg requires prompt admission to the maternity unit. Watery vaginal loss also needs careful assessment. Liquor has a distinct smell and is clear or may be stained with meconium. It can be distinguished from urine, which is yellow. Women should be advised to wear a sanitary towel if they experience any vaginal loss so that it can be closely observed and to speak to a midwife for advice.

It is normal for women to have a white vaginal discharge (leucorrhoea) during pregnancy that is heavier than when not pregnant. However, it should not be coloured, offensive or cause the woman any discomfort.

Micturition

Women should be asked if they are experiencing any problems associated with passing urine. It is abnormal for a woman to experience pain during micturition, and this may be a sign of urinary tract infection. Women who report such pain should be asked for a midstream specimen of urine, which should be sent to the laboratory for culture and sensitivity. Women often experience frequency of micturition during pregnancy because of the close proximity of the expanding uterus and bladder in early pregnancy and the pressure of the fetal head in the third trimester. It is also common for women to experience some stress incontinence during pregnancy. This can be embarrassing and difficult for women to discuss. They should be reassured that they can help improve the tone of the pelvic floor by undertaking regular pelvic floor exercises (Boyle et al 2012); however, further research is required to evaluate the long-term efficacy of pelvic floor muscle training.

Bowel function

Many pregnant women experience some alteration in their normal bowel habit when pregnant. The effect of progesterone on the smooth muscle of the bowel, further impeded by the gravid uterus, can lead to infrequent evacuation. Advice should include increasing water intake, eating additional fresh fruit and vegetables and eating a high-fibre breakfast. Keeping active is also beneficial. If the woman is taking iron tablets, it may be worth trying a different form. NICE (2008, 2017) recommends a change of diet as the first line of action. Aperients are only prescribed if these remedies fail and should be of the bulk laxative variety (Jordan 2010). The next option is an osmotic laxative such as lactulose: a study examining general practitioner prescribing for constipation (Shafe et al 2011) suggests that macrogol is gaining in popularity, increasing from 13% in 2005 to 32% in 2009. Haemorrhoids are exacerbated by constipation and may require treatment; the passage of hard stools will aggravate the haemorrhoids and the pain will make the woman reluctant to go to the toilet, thus worsening the constipation.

Dietary intake

The midwife should follow up women who were experiencing nausea and vomiting at booking. It is often assumed that once into the third trimester, this distressing symptom of pregnancy will have resolved. Unfortunately, this is not always the case, and some women vomit throughout the pregnancy. Urinalysis for ketones is useful to ensure that the problem is not causing ketosis, which can make the woman feel even worse. Kind words and compassion go a long way to helping women cope, and reassurance that the baby is not in danger is important.

Although weighing is not a routine aspect of antenatal care (NICE 2008, 2017), some women value being able to monitor their weight during pregnancy. There is evidence from an American study (Baugh et al 2016) that excessive gestational weight gain independently predicts maternal hypertension, excessive birth weight and a longer infant hospital stay.

Up to 80% of women suffer from heartburn in pregnancy (Law et al 2010), which can be painful, frequent and debilitating. Women will need advice about prevention, especially regarding keeping an upright posture and avoiding spicy foods and large meals before bedtime. Symptoms can be alleviated with prescribed antacids (remember there is no charge for prescriptions for pregnant women in the UK), although there is limited robust evidence regarding the effectiveness of pharmacology or alternative therapies such as acupuncture (Phupong & Hanprasertpong 2015).

Skin integrity

Abdominal palpation to assess fetal growth is part of each antenatal examination (see Chapter 9). This provides the midwife with the opportunity to observe the integrity of the skin and identify any areas of concern. For example, the woman may have developed stretch marks (striae gravidarum), which can be red and intensely irritating. The woman can be reassured that they will fade over time, but unfortunately never completely disappear. The use of over-the-counter preparations can help minimize the appearance of these marks, but there is no evidence that they can be prevented. The action of rubbing cream into affected areas will enhance the circulation and help keep the skin supple. Some women complain of intense itching during pregnancy. Where this is not associated with stretch marks or an obvious skin condition, this should be investigated to rule out obstetric cholestasis. Where itching is leading to intense scratching and sleepless nights, in the absence of a rash, blood should be taken for liver function tests and bile acid levels to rule out this condition (Royal College of Obstetricians and Gynaecologists (RCOG) 2011). For a summary of activities related to monitoring maternal wellbeing, see Box 5.1.

Box 5.1 Monitoring maternal wellbeing during pregnancy

- Inquire about mood
  Rationale: To identify women in need of additional support or specialist input.
  Take action if: feelings of hopelessness, self-harm, tokophobia, agitation, anxiety, obsessive thoughts
- Inquire about general activity
  Rationale: To identify women with depressed mood, debilitating fatigue or physical pain in need of further investigation.
  Take action if: agoraphobia, inertia, extreme lethargy, pelvic pain

Continued

Box 5.1 Monitoring maternal wellbeing during pregnancy *(Continued)*

- Inquire about sleep patterns
  Rationale: To identify poor quality/quantity of sleep and offer advice.
  Take action if: insomnia, narcosis
- Blood pressure measurement
  Rationale: To confirm that blood pressure remains within safe parameters. Opportunity to give advice regarding action to take if signs or symptoms of pre-eclampsia arise.
  Take action if: systolic pressure above 140 mm Hg and/or diastolic pressure above 90 mm Hg, proteinurea, headaches, epigastric pain, visual disturbances
- Urinalysis
  Rationale: To exclude the presence of protein. To detect infection or pre-eclampsia. Opportunity to give advice regarding action to take if signs or symptoms arise.
  Take action if: proteinurea, haematurea
- Leg examination
  Rationale: To identify varicose veins or deep vein thrombosis. To monitor and advise regarding oedema. Opportunity to offer advice and referral if necessary.
  Take action if: different-sized calves; hot, red areas; painful or swollen veins
- Carbon monoxide monitoring
  Rationale To identify women exposed to this poisonous gas
  Take action if: woman smokes – refer to local stop smoking support services
- Blood tests
  Rationale: To detect and treat anaemia. To detect development of rhesus antibodies.
  Take action if: results outside normal parameters, depending on local policy
- Inquire about any vaginal loss
  Rationale: To detect possible infection, premature rupture of fetal membranes or placental separation. Opportunity to give advice regarding action to take if signs or symptoms arise.
  Take action if: blood loss; loss of liquor; offensive, itchy or discolored vaginal discharge
- Inquire about bowel function
  Rationale: To identify need for dietary advice or side effects from iron therapy. Opportunity to offer preventive advice.
  Take action if: constipation, diarrhoea, haemorrhoids
- Inquire about bladder function
  Rationale: To detect infection and offer advice regarding pelvic floor exercises.
  Take action if: dysurea, incontinence
- Inquire about dietary intake
  Rationale: To identify women with eating disorders, nausea and vomiting, poor nutrition or depression. Opportunity to offer advice.
  Take action if: bulimia, anorexia, malnutrition

REFLECTION ON THE TRIGGER SCENARIO

Look back on the trigger scenario.

> *Joanna is now 25 weeks pregnant. She has just returned from her antenatal checkup with the midwife. It was not the same midwife who had taken her booking history, but she was friendly and took time to read through Jo's records. The midwife said that her blood pressure was up a bit, but when she retook it later it was fine. Jo had meant to ask her midwife what she should take for heartburn, but did not get the chance. She will call in at the chemist on her way to work.*

The scenario highlights that women do not always see the same midwife throughout their pregnancy. This lack of continuity can be a source of dissatisfaction for some women, particularly when they have a complex history that they need to retell to numerous individuals. However, if the midwife is able to take time to get to know the woman, is respectful and listens attentively to the woman's story, the consultation can be a positive experience and mutually satisfying. Now that you are familiar with the physical examination of the mother during pregnancy, you should have an insight into how the scenario relates to the evidence. The jigsaw model will now be used to explore the trigger scenario in more depth.

Effective communication

The midwife took time to read Jo's notes and get to know her, even though she had not met her before and may not meet her again. Annual and study leave, sickness and part-time working can interfere with the best intentions to provide continuity of care for women. Questions that arise from the scenario might include the following: Where was the midwife who had undertaken the booking history? How can the midwife ensure that the details of the appointment are accurately conveyed to Jo's named midwife and to Jo? What forms of communication are used between professionals antenatally?

Woman-centred care

It is evident from the scenario that Jo liked the midwife and felt relaxed and respected. She had received some feedback about her blood pressure but this was rather vague. Questions that arise from the scenario might include the following: Did the midwife convey the actual blood pressure readings to Jo? Did Jo understand what the implications of raised blood pressure might have been? Did the midwife give any advice to Jo about what to do if she experienced any potential signs of pre-eclampsia? Did

Jo leave the appointment feeling involved in her care? Jo had meant to ask about her heartburn but did not get the chance – how could this situation have been different?

Using best evidence

Raised blood pressure is a potential sign of pre-eclampsia, a condition with serious implications. It is essential that antenatal care is based on the best available evidence to detect and treat this life-threatening condition. Questions that arise from the scenario might include the following: What is the evidence to support the use of Korotkoff V as the diastolic blood pressure reading to record? Why did the midwife take Jo's blood pressure again? What is the most effective treatment for indigestion in pregnancy? What non-pharmacological measures can be taken to treat indigestion? How do midwives access evidence-based guidelines to support their practice?

Professional and legal issues

The midwife was able to convey a demeanour that enabled Jo to feel confident in her hands. Questions that arise from the scenario might include the following: How did the midwife instil Jo with trust? What action does the midwife take to ensure that her practice remains up to date? Why is it essential to maintain legible, accurate records after each antenatal appointment? What action should the midwife take if she detects raised blood pressure in a woman during an antenatal clinic visit? How does the Nursing and Midwifery (NMC) Code support effective antenatal care?

Team working

The midwife works as an autonomous practitioner within a team of healthcare professionals. She is the expert in the care of healthy pregnant women. Questions that arise from the scenario might include the following: Who can the community midwife call on if she detects an abnormality in a woman's pregnancy? How are relationships fostered and enhanced within the primary healthcare team? What processes are in place to ensure that general practitioners keep up to date with changes in protocols and guidelines? What is the role of the maternity care assistant in the care of pregnant women where you work? Which allied healthcare professionals contribute to the maternity care team?

Clinical dexterity

During the antenatal examination the midwife detected an elevation in Jo's blood pressure. Developing and maintaining this clinical skill is an essential part of the midwife's repertoire. Questions that arise from the scenario might include the following: What equipment is used in the community setting to measure blood pressure? Does the equipment in the hospital differ from that used in the hospital? Which arm should the midwife use to measure blood pressure? When was the sphygmomanometer last re-calibrated? How often should this be undertaken?

Models of care

Midwife-led care is the most appropriate model of care for women experiencing uncomplicated pregnancy. However, some women wish to have consultant-led care. Questions that arise from the scenario might include the following: Was Jo given a choice regarding the model of care she receives? Does she have a named midwife who has overall responsibility for her care? Does the midwife modify the schedule of care in light of Jo's temporary raised blood pressure? Is there an audit of which professional is the lead carer for low-risk women? What models of maternity care are available where you work?

Safe environment

The midwife detected an abnormality in Jo's blood pressure. She continued to care for Jo, undertaking the rest of her examination, before repeating the blood pressure measurement. She did not detect that Jo was suffering from heartburn. Questions that arise from the scenario might include the following: Is there sufficient flexibility in the maternity care system to spend extra time with women who need it? Was the clinic particularly busy that day? What must a midwife do if she feels that the environment of care is putting women at risk? Why did Jo not get the chance to ask about her heartburn? Are over-the-counter indigestion remedies safe for pregnant women? What dietary advice could be offered to Jo to help her manage heartburn without medication?

Promotes health

Antenatal care provides an ideal opportunity to discuss healthy lifestyle practices that can influence the health of women and their families beyond this pregnancy. Questions that arise from the scenario might include the following: Did the midwife ask Jo if she had her blood pressure checked before she was pregnant? Did she inform Jo of the actual blood pressure reading so that Jo could take an active part in noting fluctuation in this measurement? If Jo had disclosed that she had troublesome heartburn, what advice might the midwife have offered?

Further scenarios

The following scenarios enable you to consider how specific situations influence the care the midwife provides. Use the jigsaw model to explore the issues raised in the scenario.

Tracey is 36 weeks pregnant with her second baby. She has noticed that her feet and ankles are beginning to swell at the end of the day. This had not happened during her first pregnancy, and she asks the midwife if there is anything she can take to get rid of the fluid. She comments that her auntie takes 'water tablets' for swollen legs.

Practice point

Many women experience mild to moderate swelling of their hands, feet and ankles towards the end of their pregnancy and this is physiological. It is caused by a combination of increased circulating volume and impeded venous return. Symptoms are often worse during hot weather and if the woman stands for long periods. The swelling should ease overnight. Any sudden swelling, especially if associated with headache, visual disturbances or epigastric pain, should prompt the midwife to exclude the development of pre-eclampsia by taking her blood pressure and testing her urine for protein.

Further questions specific to Scenario 1 include:
1. Why do some women experience oedema during pregnancy?
2. Is oedema more prevalent in women expecting their second baby?
3. What practical advice can the midwife offer?
4. When will the oedema resolve?
5. Does the woman need referral to another health professional?
6. Are 'water tablets' prescribed for oedema in pregnancy?

Genevieve has had an uneventful pregnancy so far. She is now 35 weeks pregnant with her first baby. However, the last couple of nights' sleep have been disturbed with particularly itchy hands and feet, which she cannot stop scratching. Her mum recalls experiencing something similar when she was pregnant, but she does not remember anyone taking a great deal of notice at the time.

Practice point

Itching in pregnancy can be benign (e.g. related to stretch mark development) or a symptom of obstetric cholestasis. Severe itching should be investigated to exclude this condition, and this includes taking blood to test liver function and ascertain bile acid levels.

Further questions specific to Scenario 2 include:
1. What are the possible causes of itching during pregnancy?
2. What are the risks of obstetric cholestasis for the mother and baby?
3. How is obstetric cholestasis diagnosed?
4. How is obstetric cholestasis usually monitored?
5. How is obstetric cholestasis usually managed?

Conclusion

Women may experience a range of emotions and physical changes throughout pregnancy. The student needs to adopt a thorough, yet not intrusive, approach to antenatal health monitoring, aiming to provide personal and respectful care. She or he will assess all aspects of maternal wellbeing during the antenatal check, maximizing opportunities to promote health and take further agreed action where altered health is observed.

Resources

Mother's blood test to check her unborn baby's blood group
http://hospital.blood.co.uk/media/27899/inf1263-11-mothers-blood-test-to
-check-her-unborn-babys-blood-group.pdf
Action on pre-eclampsia: http://action-on-pre-eclampsia.org.uk
Confidential Enquiry into Maternal Deaths in the UK (Saving Lives, Improving
Mothers' Care) MBRRACE-UK 2016: https://www.npeu.ox.ac.uk/downloads/
files/mbrrace-uk/reports/MBRRACE-UK%20Maternal%20Report%202016%20
-%20website.pdf
Smoking in pregnancy – Very Brief Advice online training. National Centre for
Smoking Cessation Training. http://www.ncsct.co.uk/index.php
NHS Direct information about varicose veins: http://www.nhsdirect.nhs.uk/articles/
article.aspx?ArticleID5387#
Obstetric Cholestasis Support Website: http://www.icpsupport.org
Pelvic floor exercises: http://www.continence-foundation.org.uk
Women's Experiences of Maternity Care in the NHS in England: https://www
.npeu.ox.ac.uk/downloads/files/reports/Safely%20delivered%20NMS%20
2014.pdf
RCM public health model: https://www.rcm.org.uk/new-resources-available-for
-stepping-up-to-public-health

References

Baston, H., Hall, J., 2017. Midwifery Essentials: Basics, second ed. Elsevier, London.
Baugh, N., Harris, D., Aboueissa, A., et al., 2016. The Impact of Maternal Obesity
and Excessive Gestational Weight Gain on Maternal and Infant Outcomes in
Maine: Analysis of Pregnancy Risk Assessment Monitoring System Results
from 2000 to 2010. J. Pregnancy 10, doi:10.1155/2016/5871313.

Boyle, R., Hay-Smith, E.J.C., Cody, J.D., et al., 2012. Pelvic floor muscle training for prevention and treatment of urinary and faecal incontinence in antenatal and postnatal women. Cochrane Database Syst Rev (10), Art. No.: CD007471, doi:10.1002/14651858.CD007471.pub2.

Boyle, S., Thomas, H., Brooks, F., 2016. Women's views on partnership working with midwives during pregnancy and childbirth. Midwifery 32, 21–29.

Dowswell, T., Carroli, G., Duley, L., et al., 2015. Alternative versus standard packages of antenatal care for low-risk pregnancy. Cochrane Database Syst Rev (7), Art. No.: CD000934, doi:10.1002/14651858.CD000934.pub3.

Harding, K., Jagannathan, V., Laura Magee, L., et al., 2016. Caring for women with hypertensive disease in pregnancy. In: Knight, M., Nair, M., Tuffnell, D., et al. on behalf of MBRRACE-UK (Eds.), 2016. Saving Lives, Improving Mothers' Care - Surveillance of Maternal Deaths in the UK 2012-14 and Lessons Learned to Inform Maternity Care from the UK and Ireland Confidential Enquiries into Maternal Deaths and Morbidity 2009-14. National Perinatal Epidemiology Unit, University of Oxford, Oxford.

Jordan, S., 2010. Pharmacology for Midwives: The Evidence Base for Safe Practice, second ed. Palgrave, Basingstoke.

Knight, M., Nair, M., Tuffnell, D., et al. on behalf of MBRRACE-UK (Eds.), 2016. Saving Lives, Improving Mothers' Care - Surveillance of Maternal Deaths in the UK 2012-14 and Lessons Learned to Inform Maternity Care from the UK and Ireland Confidential Enquiries into Maternal Deaths and Morbidity 2009-14. National Perinatal Epidemiology Unit, University of Oxford, Oxford.

Law, R., Maltepe, C., Bozzo, P., et al., 2010. Treatment of heartburn and acid reflux associated with nausea and vomiting during pregnancy. Can. Fam. Physician 56 (2), 143–144.

NCSCT. National Centre for Smoking Cessation and Training, 2014. Very Brief Advice training module. [online]. Available from: http://www.ncsct.co.uk/publication_very-brief-advice.php. (Accessed 4 August 2017).

National Institute for Health and Care Excellence (NICE 2008, updated 2017). Antenatal care for uncomplicated pregnancies. CG62. https://www.nice.org.uk/guidance/cg62. (Accessed 28 October 2017).

National Institute for Health and Care Excellence (NICE 2010a, updated 2011). Hypertension in pregnancy: diagnosis and management. https://www.nice.org.uk/guidance/cg107. (Accessed 25 July 2017).

National Institute for Health and Care Excellence (NICE 2010b). Smoking: stopping in pregnancy and after childbirth. Public health guideline [PH26]. https://www.nice.org.uk/guidance/ph26. (Accessed 11 October 2017).

National Institute for Health and Care Excellence (NICE 2013). Smoking: acute, maternity and mental health services. Public health guideline [PH48]. https://www.nice.org.uk/guidance/ph48/chapter/1-Recommendations#recommendation-4-provide-intensive-support-for-people-using-maternity-services. (Accessed 11 October 2017).

National Maternity Review, 2016. Better Births. Improving outcomes of maternity services in England. Available at: https://www.england.nhs.uk/wp-content/uploads/2016/02/national-maternity-review-report.pdf.

Nursing and Midwifery Council, 2015. The code: professional standards of practice and behaviour for nurses and midwives. https://www.nmc.org.uk/globalassets/sitedocuments/nmc-publications/nmc-code.pdf.

Phupong, V., Hanprasertpong, T., 2015. Interventions for heartburn in pregnancy. Cochrane Database Syst Rev (9), Art. No.: CD011379, doi:10.1002/14651858. CD011379.pub2.

RCOG, 2011. Obstetric cholestasis. Green top guideline No. 43. https://www .rcog.org.uk/globalassets/documents/guidelines/gtg_43.pdf. (Accessed 26 July 2017).

Redshaw, M., Henderson, J., 2015. Safely delivered: a national survey of women's experience of maternity care 2014. Oxford. https://www.npeu.ox.ac.uk/ downloads/files/reports/Safely%20delivered%20NMS%202014.pdf.

Shafe, A., Lee, S., Dalrymple, J., et al., 2011. The LUCK study: Laxative Usage in patients with GP-diagnosed Constipation in the UK, within the general population and in pregnancy. An epidemiological study using the General Practice Research Database (GPRD). Therap. Adv. Gastroenterol 4 (6), 343–363. doi :10.1177/1756283X11417483.

WHO, 2016. Recommendations on Antenatal Care for a Positive Pregnancy Experience. World Health Organization. http://apps.who.int/iris/bitstream/ 10665/250796/1/9789241549912-eng.pdf?ua=1.

CHAPTER 6

Monitoring women's emotional wellbeing in the antenatal period

TRIGGER SCENARIO

Simone, a community-based midwife, rings Joanna's doorbell. This is Joanna's first pregnancy and she is now 28 weeks pregnant. Joanna eventually opens the door. 'Hello', Simone says. At which point Joanna bursts into tears. 'I am so scared', she sobs.

Introduction

The onset of pregnancy will be a time of great joy for many women and their families. It will be a fulfilment of something that has been hoped for and wanted and a positive event in a woman's life. For other women a pregnancy may bring more negative emotions, especially in situations where it is unexpected or unplanned. However, most women will find that there will be a mixture of emotions over the course of the pregnancy, as it is a powerful, life-changing experience that affects the woman and those who are close to her. In an holistic approach to care it is important to think about the time of pregnancy in a complete way. How a woman will react in pregnancy will depend on many factors, including her experiences before she became pregnant. Care will entail recognition of what is a natural emotional reaction to pregnancy in contrast to recognizing when reactions are pathological.

The World Health Organization (WHO 2014) defines mental health as:

> *A state of well-being in which every individual realizes his or her own potential, can cope with the normal stresses of life, can work productively and fruitfully, and is able to make a contribution to her or his community.*

Part of the role of the midwife is to help women try to achieve this state. Swinton (2001:35) has identified seven elements that define mental health:

+ Absence of illness
+ Appropriate social behaviour

+ Freedom from worry and guilt
+ Personal competence and control
+ Self-acceptance and self-actualization
+ Unification and organization of personality
+ Open-mindedness and flexibility

Emotional and mental wellbeing should be considered in an holistic way, recognizing the continuum between the body, mind and spirit (Clarke 2013). This means that what affects the physical part of a person will affect the other parts and vice versa.

Activity

Think about yourself. How do you feel in relation to the seven elements listed? Consider the list and relate it to the pregnant women in your care. Which elements are relevant to them at this time?

The aim of this chapter is to consider emotional wellbeing in relation to pregnancy and to enable a midwife to provide women with support as they experience different emotions.

Background

Pregnancy is a time of change and adjustment. The changes that take place are physical, in that the fetus will be growing inside a woman and affecting her bodily processes. Mullin (2002:38) writes that:

> At no other time will an otherwise healthy adult undergo such widespread, rapid and undesired change in the shape and size of her body.

The changes will also be psychological, as she goes through adaptation into being a mother of this child (Jomeen 2017; Rubin 1984). The profound nature of this change leads women to consider the experience as meaningful and spiritual (Lundgren 2017). It is important to recognize how the physical changes that take place in pregnancy can affect the emotional moods of women and how psychological changes may also present with physical symptoms.

Activity

Remind yourself of the menstrual cycle and the changes in hormonal function in pregnancy. How does your mood change throughout your menstrual cycle?

Hormonal influences

During pregnancy there are changes in circulating hormones to maintain the developing fetus. In the early weeks of pregnancy human chorionic gonadotrophin is produced before the development of the placenta. Over the pregnancy the levels of oestrogens and progesterone rise with a subsequent effect on other normally produced hormones. Though a significant amount of research has been carried out on the effects of these hormones on mood, their impact is particularly manifest when they are combined with effects of stress, lack of social support and anxiety (Biaggi et al 2016). There is also evidence to show that stress in pregnancy has some effect on the immune system and consequently may affect the growth and development of the fetus (Brunton 2013).

Physical changes

> **Activity**
>
> Ask someone who has had a baby (or consider this if you have) what they felt about the changes that were taking place in their body. Find out more about the emotional impact of common pregnancy symptoms such as nausea and vomiting, fatigue and labile mood.

Physical changes take place in women over pregnancy, such as expanding waist lines and increase in hip, thigh and breast size. In addition, women may experience changes to eyesight, skin pigment, blood pressure and breathing. Women may experience symptoms over the pregnancy of nausea or vomiting, fatigue, backache, heartburn, oedema or urinary or bowel changes that may have an influence on her feelings about herself. Certainly, poor sleep quality in early pregnancy has been linked with antenatal depression (Zsamboky 2017). Physical illness in pregnancy, such as anaemia, hyperemesis gravidarum or a thyroid condition, may lead to symptoms that mirror those of depression, or may lead to signs of low mood if the problem is not identified (Timms 2016).

Body image

Changing identity during pregnancy also entails dealing with a changing body image (Breda et al 2015). A woman's view of her body image before pregnancy will be related to her cultural views and the society in which she lives. For some women being pregnant and growing in size will make them feel happiness and positive thoughts related to meaning of the experience (Modh et al 2011). For others they may feel more negative about these changes (Hodgkinson et al 2014). The complexity of the portrayal of the ideal body and the introduction of social media have added to the negative views. It has been shown that use of social media has an impact on women's body image (Hicks & Brown 2017). Yet this is in a context where weight in the population is increasing. It is being recognized that poor body image and relationship with food for the mother will subsequently affect the infant (Orbach & Rubin 2014). Poor body image in pregnancy has also been linked to a shorter time breastfeeding (Brown et al 2015). Poor body image and poor self-esteem are linked, and this may then be expressed through excessive dieting or purging of the body (Lavender 2007). There is gathering evidence that poor nutritional status may have an influence on psychological wellbeing in adults (Serci 2008) and vice versa (Jung et al 2017). Exploration of a woman's diet in pregnancy should be made, especially if she has a low mood status.

Sexuality

The physical changes of the woman are also linked to her views of her sexual self. Price (1988:31) writes:

> Pregnancy is a clear label both that the person is a woman and that she is sexually active.

Her changing physical shape means that she is recognized by others as a sexual being (Mullin 2002:39). Pregnancy leads to changes of status in society with recognition that where she has previously been a daughter, she is now becoming a mother. This may be a complex state, particularly for some women who may feel uncomfortable about displaying their sexual selves and may choose to hide being pregnant for as long as possible. For others being pregnant may heighten their sexual feelings, whereas others may experience a lowered libido (Jones et al 2011).

Stewart (2004:33) writes:

> …women's bodies are likely to be touched more during and immediately after pregnancy than at any other time.

A woman's concepts of her body and acceptance of being touched by 'strangers' will be linked to her emotional wellbeing in pregnancy. More intensive aversion to being touched may be felt by women who are currently, or have been, in an abusive relationship. It could have a detrimental effect on women's mental health, and they will need specialist support, alongside careful midwifery care (Baird 2007; Gutteridge 2009).

> **Activity**
>
> Think about how you feel about being touched by strangers. Having reflected on this, in what way could you enhance your practice to enable the women you look after to feel better about this? Think about how a woman may respond to your touch if she has previously experienced any form of an abusive relationship.

Psychological changes

Significant psychological changes occur in women and their partners over the course of pregnancy. Complex processes take place in relationships between partners and their wider family as they adjust to the impending addition of a new family member (Raphael-Leff 2005; Raynor & England 2010). Women's expectations and previous experiences of pregnancy will have a significant effect on how she copes and adapts to the changes that take place. These may be influenced by many factors, including how she has been brought up, the society and culture in which she resides and the social support she receives.

The process of adaptation often begins before pregnancy when couples make the decision to have a child. The reasons for this will be individual to the people involved, and sometimes will be subconscious (Bergum 1989; Raphael-Leff 2005). For women who were not expecting pregnancy, the process of adaptation may take longer as they have to come to terms with the news (Steinberg & Rubin 2014). Women who are experiencing a complicated pregnancy or have had a previous pregnancy loss may take a longer time to build a relationship with their unborn child until the risk or threat to the pregnancy has passed or they have passed the anniversary of the loss (Mills et al 2014).

Spirituality

Within an holistic philosophy of care, it is essential to consider the relevance of spirituality to the woman (Crowther & Hall 2015). Pregnancy and childbirth is considered to be a powerful and meaningful event, which is a rite of passage into motherhood (Moloney 2007). Spiritual and religious beliefs may become more significant during pregnancy, with these providing a source of coping with stressful situations (Carver & Ward 2007; Jesse et al 2007; Price et al 2007). The Royal College of Psychiatrists recognizes the significance of thinking about the spiritual dimension in relation to mental wellbeing (2014). Spiritual care could lead to:

+ Better self-control, self-esteem and confidence
+ Faster and easier recovery (often through healthy grieving of losses and through recognizing their strengths)
+ Better relationships – with self, others and God/creation/nature

+ A new sense of meaning, hope and peace of mind. This has enabled them to accept and live with continuing problems or to make changes where possible

This signifies that aiming to provide a spiritual focus to care may help women with emotional needs during pregnancy. The midwife may establish women's spiritual need by asking appropriate questions in the antenatal period (Hall 2010) and staying alert to signs of distress.

Sources of stress

Maternity provision in the UK includes many opportunities for women to make 'informed choices' (The National Maternity Review 2016). Such choices include place of birth, choice of caregiver and antenatal screening methods, but they do not always come without a cost. It has been suggested that the introduction of screening may lead to psychological distress (Harris et al 2012). Sherr (1995) sums that up in relation to antenatal screening:

+ May cause anxiety
+ Delay in feedback may cause 'adverse emotional consequences'
+ Poor communication skills may raise anxiety
+ Anxiety may remain even after the outcomes have been negative or positive
+ Medical practitioners are poor at identifying the nature of anxiety in women
+ Widespread programmes make it difficult to respond to individual need and concern

Women may also experience grief and loss as they may lose some part of their identity through changing roles (Mercer 1995). This grief may be in relation to loss of status in leaving employment. It is common that women will express feelings of ambivalence, of 'not being ready' to have a baby during pregnancy, even if they have made a choice to become pregnant (Raphael-Leff 2005). They now need to adjust to their new identity:

> We can relate the change from non-mother to mother as a form of loss where women may have to reinterpret the ways in which they view themselves in accordance with their new role as a mother and caregiver, and reevaluate their former self, as well as adjust to their new identity which is now on view to the wider society.
>
> (Atkinson 2006)

Activity

Think about your current experience of giving information about antenatal screening tests and being with women receiving results. In light of the earlier information, are there ways this could be improved?

Tokophobia

Many women will experience anxiety at some point over pregnancy; however, Lorraine Sherr (1995:137) suggests that anxiety may be a 'protective positive emotion' as a result of stressors. Problems may only arise should the anxiety be out of proportion to the stressors. Fears and anxieties relating to the wellbeing of the growing fetus are common. A pathological condition of intense fear has been defined and labelled *tokophobia* (Hofberg & Ward 2004), though Denis Walsh (2002) has challenged whether this is actually a 'normal' reaction to a traumatic event.

Hofberg and Ward (2003) state there are different types of tokophobia:

+ Primary – when women have not had a baby before
+ Secondary – where women have had previous traumatic deliveries
+ Secondary to depressive illness in pregnancy

The prevalence of tokophobia varies considerably between countries; in the BIDENS study of 7200 women in six European countries, it ranged from 1.9% to 14.2% (Van Parys et al 2012). Tokophobia is more common in women in their first pregnancy, but women who experience a traumatic birth are five times more likely to fear their next birth (Storksen et al 2013).

> **Activity**
>
> Think about the three types of tokophobia described by Hofberg and Ward. As a midwife, how would you support women in these situations?

Antenatal depression

Understanding of mental wellbeing has often been focused on the postnatal period of childbirth rather than before birth. However, it has been identified that around 12% of women experience a type of antenatal depression, with 13% experiencing anxiety and many experience both (National Institute for Health and Care Excellence (NICE) 2016). Pre-existing psychiatric disorders may become worse in pregnancy (Hadwin 2007; Weeks 2007).

In Raymonds' (2009) study of some women's experience of antenatal depression, it was identified that some found it hard to reveal their feelings and that it was common to feel 'emotional isolation'. The author concluded this could have been helped through provision of continuity of carer. The author further established that the partner may also have needs for support. The women identified helpful support mechanisms: massage, social groups, practical skill development and exercise plus access to web-based support groups.

In a systematic review (Biaggi et al 2016) it has been identified that the most significant factors leading to antenatal depression were:

- The lack of partner or of social support
- A history of abuse or of domestic abuse
- A personal history of mental illness
- An unplanned or unwanted pregnancy
- Adverse events in life and high perceived stress
- Present or past pregnancy complications
- Pregnancy loss

Difficult social situations that need to be considered include domestic violence, which may have a significant effect on the emotional wellbeing of the pregnant woman (Baird 2007). It should also be recognized that mental ill health will have a long-term effect on the child (O'Donnell et al 2014).

The best treatment for antenatal depression is not clear. A Cochrane review of psychosocial and psychological interventions (Dennis & Dowswell 2013) identified various strategies but concluded that evidence is insufficient to provide a recommendation. National guidance (NICE 2014, 2017) highlights the need to discuss the risk and benefits of potential harmful medication alongside those of psychological intervention, in order to make appropriate choices.

Activity

With this knowledge on antenatal depression, how could maternity services be adapted to improve care of women? What sort of information should the midwife find out?

National guidance

Mental health services and care is a high priority for the UK government. The most recent 5-year review for services held eight principles for improving services, and these can be applied to maternity care (Mental Health Task Force 2016):

- Decisions must be locally led
- Care must be based on the best available evidence
- Services must be designed in partnership with people who have mental health problems and with carers
- Inequalities must be reduced to ensure all needs are met, across all ages
- Care must be integrated – spanning people's physical, mental and social needs

- Prevention and early intervention must be prioritized
- Care must be safe, effective and personal and delivered in the least restrictive setting
- The right data must be collected and used to drive and evaluate progress

Midwives have a health promotion focus that requires them to consider how positive mental health may be supported in pregnancy (Hall 2007). Further, midwives should be able to recognize the needs of women with mental health challenges and be able to refer to relevant services. The NICE (2014, 2017) guidelines give information on appropriate assessment of mental health conditions in pregnancy. Advice is also given about referral systems.

Activity

Access these guidelines from the NICE web pages and consider the relevance of the information to emotional health. Think about how they apply to the women in your care:

https://www.nice.org.uk/guidance/cg192/chapter/recommendations#assessment-and-care-planning-in-pregnancy-and-the-postnatal-period

---

Professional regulation

The role of a midwife with regard to emotional health is clearly stated in UK midwifery standards of competence:

> [A]ct on their understanding of psychological, social, emotional and spiritual factors that may positively or adversely influence normal physiology, and be competent in applying this in practice.
>
> (Nursing and Midwifery Council (NMC) 2017:4)

Midwives need to have knowledge of the risk factors for poor mental health in pregnancy and how to identify them (Rothera & Oates 2011). They also have clear responsibility to refer to other professionals when the circumstances are outside their scope of practice of normal childbirth.

Student midwives are expected to learn to:

> …undertake critical decision-making to support appropriate referral of either the woman or baby to other health professionals or agencies when there is recognition of normal processes being adversely affected and compromised.
>
> (NMC 2017)

The standards for education also have essential skills where students should learn to:

> Support the creation and maintenance of environments that promote the health, safety and wellbeing of women, babies and others.
>
> (p. 33)

Midwives' role in mental health assessment

Consideration should be given to the environment where antenatal care takes place (Newburn 2006) to ensure women feel safe to disclose sensitive information – this has been highlighted by NICE (2008, 2017). To establish the needs of women, midwives should assess them appropriately. Asking the 'right' questions and providing continual assessment through developing a relationship over pregnancy is the ideal situation. Continuity of care may enable midwives to recognize emotional changes more quickly (Hall 2007:41). A positive mother–midwife relationship is key to facilitating information sharing (Byrom & Gaudion 2010).

Rubertsson et al's (2005) study suggests that a comprehensive 'psycho-social' history should be taken in early pregnancy that includes addressing:

+ Previous mental health problems
+ A woman's social support
+ Stressful life events
+ Employment status

NICE (2014, 2017) recommends that at the first contact with a health professional in pregnancy, women are asked the following 'Whooley questions':

+ During the past month, have you often been bothered by feeling down, depressed or hopeless?
+ During the past month, have you often been bothered by having little interest or pleasure in doing things?

More recently, NICE (2014, 2017) suggest that women be asked two items from the Generalized Anxiety Scale (GAD):

+ Over the last 2 weeks, have you been bothered by feeling nervous, anxious or on edge?
+ Over the last 2 weeks, have you been bothered by not being able to stop or control worrying?

For details how to score the GAD and suggested responses, see Table 6.1.

The answers to these questions should help midwives establish if the woman is having a 'normal' reaction to pregnancy or if there is some underlying mental health condition requiring referral. However, women may not always feel comfortable disclosing their emotional distress (Reilly

Table 6.1: Scoring the Generalized Anxiety Scale (GAD)

Over the last 2 weeks, how often have you been bothered by …	Not at all	Several days	>7 days	Nearly every day
… Feeling nervous, anxious or on edge?	0	1	2	3
… Not being able to stop or control worrying?	0	1	2	3
Total score = Action taken if total score 3 or more	3–4 Watchful waiting and review by midwife			
	5–6 Self-referral to IAPT or GP and review			

GP, General Practitioner; IAPT, Improving Access to Psychological Therapies Service

et al 2015), and some will be dissuaded by family and friends who encourage normalization of symptoms (Kingston et al 2015). Definite identification of emotional or mental health disorders can be difficult to establish.

Other mental wellbeing conditions

NICE (2014, 2017) states that women with psychiatric conditions and addictive tendencies require more specialist care. These conditions include issues such as eating disorders, drug or alcohol addiction, bipolar disorder and obsessive disorder. The midwife must acknowledge the limitations of her expertise and must always involve the wider multi-professional team in their care.

> **Activity**
>
> What services are available where you work for women who experience post-traumatic stress disorder (PTSD) after a previous birth experience? What is the role of 'birth after thoughts' services, and how can they help women in the antenatal period?

Continuing monitoring

Women should be asked about their emotional wellbeing throughout pregnancy. A woman's social circumstances may change and create extra stressors on her whilst she continues to adapt to her changing identity. She may experience physical complications or unpleasant symptoms that lead to anxiety or fear. The midwife can play an important role in alleviating unnecessary distress and providing a supportive ear when circumstances are challenging.

NICE (2014, 2017) states:

> At each antenatal appointment, healthcare professionals should offer consistent information and clear explanations, and should provide pregnant women with an opportunity to discuss issues and ask questions.

Local services and support networks may be available to women such as volunteer doula programmes or case loading schemes that can provide additional support to women with a vulnerable mental health status.

REFLECTION ON THE TRIGGER SCENARIO

Look back on the trigger scenario.

> Simone, a community-based midwife, rings Joanna's doorbell. This is Joanna's first pregnancy and she is now 28 weeks pregnant. Joanna eventually opens the door. 'Hello', Simone says. At which point Joanna bursts into tears. 'I am so scared', she sobs.

This scenario describes a specific encounter during pregnancy. With the knowledge you now have about emotional changes in pregnancy, you should be able to consider Joanna's situation and how a midwife may be able to help her. The jigsaw model will now be used to explore the situation in more depth.

Woman-centred care

Ensuring sensitive, individualized care for women means that midwives may be able to recognize when women need more intensive input from the midwife herself or from other health professionals. In this scenario the following questions could be asked: Is this a 'routine' visit or has it been instigated due to previous concerns about Joanna's wellbeing? Has she been previously included in plans about her care and asked what her needs are? Are her partner and family involved in her care? How does Joanna's experience at the moment relate to her expectations of this pregnancy? How will Simone include Joanna in the next aspects of her care?

Using best evidence

In this scenario the midwife needs to use the best evidence available to make decisions about the next aspects of her care. Questions that need to be addressed to ensure that the woman's care is evidence based include the following: What questions will Simone ask to establish what is happening to Joanna? What is the evidence around the causes of emotional distress in pregnancy? What evidence is there about appropriate forms of care or treatment? How will Simone use national guidelines to enable the most appropriate care for Joanna?

Professional and legal

Midwives should always practice within the framework of their profession and the law. In this scenario questions that need to be addressed to ensure that the woman's care fulfils statutory obligations include the following: Has Simone received enough appropriate training in relation to mental health concerns? How do the standards of practice and code of conduct help her in Joanna's care? Are there any national or international guidelines relating to Joanna's care?

Team working

Though community-based midwives often work alone, they are also based within a primary health environment that involves other health professionals. Questions that need to be addressed in this scenario are the following: Are Joanna's needs significant to warrant inviting involvement of other professionals? If so, who will this be? Where will Simone record information for other health professionals? How will Simone make contact with other health professionals if required?

Effective communication

In caring for women during the antenatal period, it is important to use appropriate communication skills, especially in relation to mental wellbeing. A midwife should especially listen to what a woman says and carefully observe her body language. Questions that may be considered in this scenario are the following: Has Simone already developed a relationship with Joanna? Does she observe Joanna to be behaving differently? What questions should Simone ask about Joanna's feelings? What clues could be obtained from what and how Joanna replies? How should Simone record the discussion?

Clinical dexterity

In relation to emotional issues clinical skills may not be usually required; however, if the midwife needs to carry out any tests after the discussion, she should use sensitivity and gentleness. Questions that could arise include the following: Does Simone need to make any clinical assessments in relation to Joanna's care? Is this the appropriate time to carry out these assessments?

Models of care

In relation to antenatal care there are currently a number of models that midwives practice in the UK. How care is organized may have a positive or negative effect on the emotional wellbeing of some women. In this situation, questions that could be raised are as follows: Does Simone work in a team of colleagues who aim to provide continuity through the whole pregnancy continuum? Would continuity be beneficial in this situation? Is home-based care more beneficial in this situation? If so, why would this be? Are other professional groups involved in the provision of the care Simone is giving?

Safe environment

All midwifery care should be carried out in a safe environment, for the woman, for her family member and for the midwife. Unpredictability of mental health issues means that midwives should be vigilant to ensure safety is maintained. Questions that could be asked about this scenario are as follows: Is Joanna in a safe environment in her home, or are there reasons to believe she may be putting herself or her family at risk? Is Simone safe in visiting Joanna at home as a lone professional?

Promotes health

Antenatal care provides many opportunities for midwives to promote the emotional health of a woman, her family and the community in which they work. In this scenario questions that could be asked to ensure that the woman's care promotes health include the following: Does the environment where Joanna is living promote her mental wellbeing? Are there issues in the home that are damaging her health? Are there ways Simone could promote Joanna's emotional health at this time?

Further scenarios

The following scenarios enable you to consider how specific situations influence the care the midwife provides. Use the jigsaw model to explore the issues raised in each situation.

SCENARIO 1

Comfort has arrived at the antenatal clinic. She is 20 weeks pregnant and has just been transferred into the area as a refugee from a war-torn African country. She has arrived with her sister and two other children. Many of her family, including her partner and parents, are still in Africa. She speaks some English but does not always understand.

Practice point

Women who arrive as refugees may have considerable emotional needs. Not only are they living in strange and often impoverished environments, but many carry emotional scars of the experiences they have had in their homeland or of the journey they have had in getting to this country. Loss of family members or long-term separation may add to their burdens. Being able to access services may also be a challenge, as they may find it hard to understand our maternity system. Language difficulties may compound understanding of needs on both sides, and midwives need to be cautious in interpreting the emotional status of the woman before them.

Further questions specific to Scenario 1 include:
1. What feelings may Comfort be experiencing?
2. What effect could these have on the pregnancy?
3. What questions may the midwife ask her about her feelings?
4. Who should the midwife ask to provide translation if required?
5. What would be the most appropriate model of care?

SCENARIO 2

Carmel, a community midwife, receives a telephone call from the antenatal clinic to say that, Anna, a woman on her caseload, has received a diagnosis of a fetal abnormality on an ultrasound. Anna intends to continue the pregnancy. Carmel promises to visit her at home.

Practice point

In a straightforward pregnancy the use of antenatal screening may cause a level of anxiety. This will be heightened should she go on to have a positive diagnostic test result. Choosing to continue pregnancy may be a difficult decision. Women and their families will need continual support in coming to terms with their fears, anxieties and grief of loss of expectations, as well as to build up a relationship with the unborn baby.

Further questions specific to Scenario 2 include:
1. What communication skills will Carmel use when she is with Anna?
2. What sorts of questions will she ask?
3. What feelings may Anna be experiencing?
4. How may the partner and family be supported in this situation?
5. What model of care will be best over the rest of the pregnancy?
6. Which other professionals may be included in Anna's care?

Conclusion

Pregnancy brings changes to all aspects of a woman's life, and in particular, significant emotional and psychological adaptations will take place. The midwife has an important role in recognizing the needs of women and helping meet those needs in a holistic way. She also should recognize when the psychological reactions are pathological and require referral to other professionals for further assessment and support.

Resources

MIND (National Association for Mental health) https://www.mind.org.uk/information-support/types-of-mental-health-problems/postnatal-depression-and-perinatal-mental-health/#.Weem8TLGxMA

Maternal Mental Health Alliance: https://maternalmentalhealthalliance.org

Maternal Mental Health – Women's Voices, Royal College of Obstetricians and Gynaecologists https://www.rcog.org.uk/en/patients/maternal-mental-health---womens-voices/

Royal College of Midwives: Maternal Emotional wellbeing and Infant Development. https://www.rcm.org.uk/sites/default/files/Emotional%20Wellbeing_Guide_WEB.pdf

Self-harm support website: http://www.harmless.org.uk

Tommy's: Mental health before, during and after pregnancy. https://www.tommys.org/pregnancy-information/im-pregnant/mental-health-during-and-after-pregnancy

References

Atkinson, B., 2006. Gaining motherhood, losing identity. MIDIRS Midwifery Digest 16 (2), 170–174.

Baird, K., 2007. Domestic abuse, violence and mental health. In: Price, S.A. (Ed.), Mental Health in Pregnancy and Childbirth. Churchill Livingstone, Edinburgh.

Bergum, V., 1989. Woman to mother: a transformation. Bergin & Garvey Publishers Inc. Massachusetts.

Biaggi, A., Conroy, S., Pawlby, S., Pariante, C.M., 2016. Identifying the women at risk of antenatal anxiety and depression: A systematic review. J. Affect. Disord. 191, 62–77. doi:10.1016/j.jad.2015.11.014.

Breda, J., Lehmann Schumann, N., Arshad, S., 2015. Body Image Pregnancy and birth. http://www.euro.who.int/__data/assets/pdf_file/0003/277734/Body-image-and-pregnancy.pdf?ua=1.

Brown, A., Rance, J., Warren, L., 2015. Body image concerns during pregnancy are associated with a shorter breastfeeding duration. Midwifery 31 (1), 80–89.

Brunton, P.J., 2013. Effects of maternal exposure to social stress during pregnancy: consequences for mother and offspring. Reproduction 146 (5), R175–R189. doi:10.1530/REP-13-0258. Print 2013.

Byrom, S., Gaudion, A., 2010. Empowering mothers: Strengthening the future. In: Byrom, S., Edwards, G., Bick, D. (Eds.), Essential Midwifery Practice Postnatal Care. Wiley-Blackwell, Chichester, pp. 95–115.

Carver, N., Ward, B., 2007. Spirituality in pregnancy: a diversity of experiences and needs. Br. J. Midwifery 15 (5), 294–296.

Clarke, J., 2013. Spiritual Care in Everyday Nursing Practice: A New Approach. Palgrave MacMillan, Basingstoke.

Crowther, S., Hall, J., 2015. Spirituality and spiritual care in and around childbirth. Women Birth 28 (2), 173–178. doi:10.1016/j.wombi.01.001.

Dennis, C.L., Dowswell, T., 2013. Interventions (other than pharmacological, psychosocial or psychological) for treating antenatal depression. Cochrane Database Syst. Rev. (7), CD006795, doi:10.1002/14651858.CD006795.pub3.

Gutteridge, K., 2009. 'From the deep' Surviving child sexual abuse into adulthood: consequences and implications for maternity services. MIDIRS Midwifery Digest 19 (1), 125–129.

Hadwin, P., 2007. Common mental health disorders. In: Price, S.A. (Ed.), Mental Health in Pregnancy and Childbirth. Churchill Livingstone, Edinburgh.

Hall, J., 2007. Promoting mental well-being. In: Price, S.A. (Ed.), Mental Health in Pregnancy and Childbirth. Churchill Livingstone, Edinburgh.

Hall, J., 2010. Spirituality and labour care. In: Walsh, D., Downe, S. (Eds.), Essential Midwifery Practice: Intrapartum Care. Blackwell, Oxford.

Harris, J.M., Franck, L., Michie, S., 2012. Assessing the psychological effects of prenatal screening tests for maternal and foetal conditions: a systematic review. J. Reprod. Infant Psychol. 30, 3.

Hicks, S., Brown, A., 2017. Higher Facebook use predicts greater body image dissatisfaction during pregnancy: The role of self-comparison. Midwifery 40, 132–140.

Hodgkinson, E., Smith, D.M., Wittkowski, A., 2014. Women's experiences of their pregnancy and postpartum body image and their transition to motherhood: A metasynthesis. BMC Pregnancy Childbirth 14, 1–11. doi:10.1186/1471-2393-14-330.

Hofberg, K., Ward, M.R., 2003. Fear of pregnancy and childbirth. Postgrad. Med. J. 79 (935), 505–510.

Hofberg, K., Ward, M.R., 2004. Fear of childbirth, tocophobia and mental health in mothers: The obstetric-psychiatric interface clinical. Obstet. Gynecol. 47 (3), 527–534.

Jesse, D.E., Schoneboom, C., Blanchard, A., 2007. The effect of faith or spirituality in pregnancy: a content analysis. J. Holist. Nurs. 25 (3), 151–158.

Jomeen, J., 2017. Psychological context of childbirth. In: MacDonald, S., Johnson, G. (Eds.), Mayes Midwifery. Elsevier, London.

Jones, C., Chan, C., Farine, D., 2011. Sex in pregnancy. CMAJ 183 (7), 815–818. http://doi.org/10.1503/cmaj.091580.

Jung, S., Bishop, A.J., Kim, M., et al., 2017. Nutritional Status of Rural Older Adults Is Linked to Physical and Emotional Health. J. Acad. Nutr. Diet. 117 (6), 851–858.

Kingston, D., Austin, M., Heaman, M., et al., 2015. Barriers and facilitators of mental health screening in pregnancy. J. Affect. Disord. 186, 350–357.

Lavender, V., 2007. Body image: change, dissatisfaction and disturbance. In: Price, S.A. (Ed.), Mental Health in Pregnancy and Childbirth. Churchill Livingstone, Edinburgh.

Lundgren, I., 2017. Spiritual questions during childbearing. In: Crowther, S., Hall, J. (Eds.), Spirituality and childbirth; meaning and care at the start of life. Routledge, Oxford.

Mental Health Task Force, 2016. The five year forward review for mental health. https://www.england.nhs.uk/wp-content/uploads/2016/02/Mental-Health-Taskforce-FYFV-final.pdf.

Mercer, R.T., 1995. Becoming a Mother: Research on Maternal Identity from RUBIN to the Present. Springer Publishing, New York.

Mills, T.A., Ricklesford, C., Cooke, A., et al., 2014. Parents' experiences and expectations of care in pregnancy after stillbirth or neonatal death: a metasynthesis. BJOG 121 (8), 943–950.

Modh, C., Lundgren, I., Bergbom, I., 2011. First time pregnant women's experiences in early pregnancy. Int. J. Qual. Stud. Health Well-Being 6 (2), doi:10.3402/qhw.v6i2.5600. http://doi.org/10.3402/qhw.v6i2.5600.

Moloney, S., 2007. Dancing with the wind: A methodological approach to researching women's spirituality around menstruation and birth. Int. J Qual. Methods 6 (1), 114–125.

Mullin, A., 2002. Pregnant bodies, pregnant minds. Feminist Theory 3 (1), 27–44.

National Maternity Review, 2016. Better Births. Improving outcomes of maternity services in England. Available at: https://www.england.nhs.uk/wp-content/uploads/2016/02/national-maternity-review-report.pdf. (Accessed 3 October 2016).

Newburn, M., 2006. Curtains for the old delivery suite. Pract. Midwife 9 (1), 12–14.

NICE 2008, 2017. Antenatal care for uncomplicated pregnancies clinical guideline. https://www.nice.org.uk/guidance/cg62.

NICE, 2016. Antenatal and postnatal mental health. https://www.nice.org.uk/guidance/qs115/chapter/Introduction.

NICE 2014, 2017. Antenatal and postnatal mental health: clinical management and service guidance. https://www.nice.org.uk/guidance/cg192/chapter/recommendations#recognising-mental-health-problems-in-pregnancy-and-the-postnatal-period-and-referral-2.

Nursing and Midwifery Council, 2017. Standards for competence for registered midwives. https://www.nmc.org.uk/globalassets/sitedocuments/standards/nmc-standards-for-competence-for-registered-midwives.pdf.

O'Donnell, K., Glover, V., Barker, E., O'Connor, T., 2014. The persisting effect of maternal mood in pregnancy on childhood psychopathology. Dev. Psychopathol. 26 (2), 393–403. doi:10.1017/S0954579414000029.

Orbach, S., Rubin, H., 2014. Two for the price of one: The impact of body image during pregnancy and after birth. https://www.gov.uk/government/uploads/system/uploads/attachment_data/file/317739/TWO_FOR_THE_PRICE_OF_ONE.pdf.

Price, J., 1988. Motherhood: what it does to your mind. Pandora Press, London.

Price, S., Lake, M., Breen, G., et al., 2007. the spiritual experience of high-risk pregnancy. JOGNN 36 (1), 63–70.

Raphael-Leff, J., 2005. Psychological processes of childbearing, fourth ed. Anna Freud centre, London.

Raymonds, J.E., 2009. 'Creating a safety net': Women's experiences of antenatal depression and their identification of helpful community support and services during pregnancy. Midwifery 25 (1), 39–49.

Raynor, M., England, C., 2010. Psychology for midwives: pregnancy, childbirth and puerperium. Open University Press, Maidenhead.

Reilly, N., Harries, D., Loxton, C., et al., 2015. The impact of routine assessment of past or current mental health on help-seeking in the perinatal period. Women Birth 27 (4), e20–e27.

Rothera, I., Oates, M., 2011. Managing perinatal mental health: A survey of practitioners' views. Br. J. Midwifery 19, 304–313.

Royal College of Psychiatrists, 2014. Spirituality and mental health. Royal College of Psychiatrists, London. http://www.rcpsych.ac.uk/mentalhealthinformation/therapies/spiritualityandmentalhealth.aspx.

Rubertsson, C., Walderstrom, U., Wickberg, B., et al., 2005. Depressive mood in early pregnancy and postpartum: prevalence and women at risk in a national Swedish sample. J. Reprod. Infant Psychol. 23 (2), 155–166.

Rubin, R., 1984. Maternal Identity and the Maternal Experience. Springer Publishing, New York.

Serci, I., 2008. Perinatal mental health: relationships with diet and nutrition The Practising Midwife 11 (4), 37–40.

Sherr, L., 1995. The Psychology of Pregnancy and Childbirth. Blackwell Science, Oxford.

Steinberg, J.R., Rubin, L.R., 2014. Psychological Aspects of Contraception, Unintended Pregnancy, and Abortion. Policy Insights Behav. Brain Sci. 1 (1), 239–247. http://doi.org/10.1177/2372732214549328.

Stewart, M., 2004. Feminisms and the body. In: Stewart, M. (Ed.), Pregnancy, Birth and Maternity Care: Feminist Perspectives. Elsevier, Oxford.

Storksen, H., Garthus-Niegel, S., Vangen, M., et al., 2013. The impact of previous birth experiences on maternal fear of childbirth. Acta Obstet. Gynecol. Scand. 92, 318–324.

Swinton, J., 2001. Spirituality in Mental Health Care: Rediscovering a Forgotten Dimension. Jessica Kingsley Publishers, London.

Timms, P., 2016. Coping with Physical Illness. Royal College of Psychiatrists, London. http://www.rcpsych.ac.uk/mentalhealthinformation/mentalhealthproblems/physicalillness/copingwithphysicalillness.aspx.

Van Parys, A., Ryding, E., Schei, B., et al., 2012. Fear of childbirth and mode of delivery in six European countries: The BIDENS study. 22nd European Congress of Obstetrics and Gynaecology (EBCOG), Book of Abstracts (S14.4).

Walsh, D., 2002. Fear of labour and birth. Br. J. Midwifery 10 (2), 78.

Weeks, N.P., 2007. Serious mental illness and the midwife. In: Price, S.A. (Ed.), Mental Health in Pregnancy and Childbirth. Churchill Livingstone, Edinburgh.

World Health Organization, 2014. Mental Health: a state of wellbeing. http://www.who.int/features/factfiles/mental_health/en/.

Zsamboky, M.L., 2017. Sleep and Pregnancy: Understanding the Importance. Int. J. Childbirth Educ. 32 (1), 22–24.

CHAPTER 7

Blood tests in pregnancy

TRIGGER SCENARIO

Joanna is now 30 weeks pregnant. She has been feeling particularly tired, and her mum suggested that she might be anaemic. Louis is rather insulted, as he prides himself on buying the best fresh ingredients from the local market; they love cooking and eat plenty of fruits and vegetables. Joanna had a full blood count taken by the community midwife who came to the flat to do her booking history.

Introduction

Pregnancy is a time when women are faced with many choices and decisions. There is a plethora of information about why various tests are being made, but it does not always reach those women who need it most. An important aspect of the student midwife's progression from novice to competent practitioner is the development of an ability to present information to women in a meaningful way that makes sense to them. As well as developing the necessary communications skills and self-awareness to approach women with confidence and competence, the student needs to feel that she or he has a firm underpinning knowledge of the facts. Being a student is challenging. Just as you thought you were getting to grips with a subject, a new dimension emerges. As you become familiar with one policy, another is produced to take its place. Change is a constant factor in professional life, but an understanding of key principles provides a stable base from which new approaches can be explored.

This chapter considers the routine blood tests offered in pregnancy (Table 7.1). Although women may be advised to undergo such blood tests, they should not be pressured or coerced. It must also be noted that some maternity units offer different tests at different times, depending on local policy and the needs of the local community. Antenatal screening for fetal abnormality, including inherited disorders, will be considered separately in Chapter 8.

Table 7.1: Routine blood tests offered during pregnancy

Blood test	Who	When
Full blood count (FBC)	All	Booking and 28 weeks
Hepatitis B virus (HBV)	All	Booking
Blood group and rhesus factor	All	Booking
Rhesus antibody screening	Rhesus-negative women	28 weeks
Red cell alloantibodies	All	Booking and 28 weeks
Syphilis (VDRL)	All	Booking
Human immunodeficiency virus (HIV)	All	Booking
Maternal serum screening for Down's, Edwards' and Patau's syndromes (see Chapter 8)	All	Combined test at 10 + 0 days–13 weeks + 6 days; Triple/ quad test 14–20 weeks
Sickle cell anaemia (see Chapter 8)	Women (or those with partners or relatives) from Africa, Mediterranean, Far/ Middle East, Asia and Caribbean	Booking
Thalassaemia (see Chapter 8)	All	Booking

Midwives involved in taking blood from pregnant women need to consider the following:

+   Occasionally some women do not want to have what are considered by professionals to be 'routine' tests. They have a right to decline. Although you have a responsibility to inform them of the consequences of their decision and to document that you have done so, take a non-judgemental approach. As a student, you must always refer any controversy or uncertainty to a registered professional.
+   Just because there is a lot of information to absorb during pregnancy does not mean that women do not want to receive it.
+   Some women have needle phobia and need to be treated with sensitivity.
+   Some women faint when they have blood taken – always ask a woman if this is the case!
+   See *Midwifery Essentials: Basics*, Chapter 9: Venepuncture, for the procedure for taking blood.

The booking history was explored in Chapter 3. It was seen that a detailed account of the woman's current health and previous medical, social and obstetric history is taken to identify potential factors that might affect the woman's or her baby's wellbeing. Taking maternal blood is another procedure that enables further risk factors to be identified or potential pathology avoided.

The sooner that these important blood tests are taken, the sooner results can be acted upon. The National Institute for Health and Care Excellence (NICE 2008, 2017) guidance recommends that the booking appointment take place by week 10 of the pregnancy. However, when blood is taken from women depends on the model of care in operation and on the local services available. Some community midwives who undertake the booking history in the community also take the booking bloods at the same time. It is important that there is a system to ensure safe transportation of these blood samples to the local laboratory, which is usually situated in the hospital trust. The midwife will often make her booking appointments in the morning so that the samples can meet the pick-up service that serves the general practitioner's surgery or health centre that she links with. Where such services do not exist, women attend the hospital for booking bloods, usually at the same time as the first scan. In some areas, the practice nurse takes blood after appropriate counselling by the midwife, and there is a local arrangement for samples to be taken at a time that coincides with other clinics.

Whoever takes the blood or requests that it is taken by someone else should ensure that the result is followed up and documented in the appropriate place.

Activity

Make sure you know what a phlebotomist is. Find out if there is a phlebotomy service at the trust where you work. Think about when women have their booking bloods taken in your locality and who normally takes them.

Blood tests in pregnancy

For a summary of the blood tests routinely offered in pregnancy, see Table 7.1.

Full blood count

The full blood count is taken to identify maternal anaemia with the aim of treating the condition, if necessary. However, it also provides a useful

Table 7.2: The full blood count in relation to pregnancy

Test	What	Normal (women)	Pregnancy
Haemoglobin (Hb)	Amount of haemoglobin in the blood measured in grams per litre (g/L)	125–155	Falls until about 30 weeks (steepest drop by 20 weeks) then rises slightly to term
Red cell count (RCC)	Number of red cells per litre of blood: 310^{12} per litre	4.2–4.5	Falls by about 1 until 30–34 weeks
Haematotcrit (Hct) of packed cell volume (PCV)	Percentage of blood cells to total blood volume	35–45	Falls by about 6% until 30 weeks then rises slightly to term
Mean corpuscular (cell) volume (MCV)	An estimated volume of individual red blood cells (fL)	80–100	Increase in macrocytic anaemia; decrease in microcytic anaemia
Mean cell haemoglobin (MCH)	Haemoglobin content within erythrocyte of average size (pg)	27–32	Increase in macrocytic anaemia; decrease in microcytic anaemia
Red cell mass	Total volume of red blood cells in the circulation	1400	Up to 1650 by term
White cell count (WCC)	Total number of white blood cells in the circulation	4–11	May be raised up to 15
Platelets	Number of platelets per litre of blood ($_310^3$) per mm^3	150–400	Slight decrease

Sources include: Chamberlain & Morgan (2002), Luckmann & Sorensen (1980), Rankin (2017), Shuttleworth (2002).

picture of the woman's current health status in many more respects (Table 7.2). For example, a fall in platelets may be seen in women who develop pre-eclampsia, and a raised white cell count may be indicative of underlying infection. In some trusts, serum ferritin levels are also measured, as they reflect the woman's iron reserves and fall before haemoglobin levels.

Iron levels are a balance between dietary intake, demand and iron loss. In pregnancy dietary intake may be similar, and there is an increased demand from the developing fetus and placenta in addition to the growth of the uterus and expanding blood volume. The woman will also lose blood at the birth and postnatally, so her pre-pregnancy status and continuing dietary intake must be sufficient to keep up with this anticipated demand and loss. The extra iron requirement is estimated to be 1000 mg (Khalafallah & Dennis 2012).

It is normal for a woman's haemoglobin to fall in pregnancy, and this reflects an expansion in plasma volume which exceeds the increase in red cell mass. A failure of the haemoglobin concentration to fall has been linked with an increase in the incidence of preterm birth and low birth weight (Steer et al 1995) and pre-eclampsia (Aghamohammadi et al 2011). Stephansson et al (2000), in a matched case-control study, found an association between high first haemoglobin and increased risk of stillbirth.

NICE (2008, 2017) recommend that a haemoglobin level of less than 110 g/L at booking and below 105 g/L at 28 weeks should be investigated and iron supplementation considered. If supplementation cannot be tolerated or there is insufficient response, parenteral iron may be considered to treat anaemia, especially if surgery is anticipated.

Activity

Find out what is meant by 'haemolytic anaemia' and 'haemorrhagic anaemia'. Make sure you can identify the signs and symptoms of iron-deficiency anaemia. Find out how much the plasma volume increases in pregnancy. Consider how anaemia is treated where you work.

Blood group and rhesus factor

The batch of blood samples taken at the booking appointment includes blood group and rhesus factor. There are four blood groups and each may be either rhesus positive or negative, giving eight different types in total (Table 7.3).

It is important to know the woman's blood group in the event that she might require an emergency blood transfusion. However, when it is anticipated that a woman might need a blood transfusion, during a caesarean section or after a postpartum haemorrhage, for example, a blood sample will be taken so that her blood and donor blood can be 'cross-matched' in the laboratory to ensure compatibility of the transfused blood with the woman's blood.

Identifying a woman's rhesus factor is important during pregnancy for the 15% of women who are rhesus negative. If blood from a rhesus-negative person mixes with blood from a rhesus-positive person, rhesus antibodies

Table 7.3: Blood groups

Group	Rhesus 1	Rhesus 2
A	A_1	A_2
B	B_1	B_2
AB	AB_1	AB_2
O	O_1	O_2

Box 7.1 Prevention of rhesus antibodies

Development of rhesus antibodies by the mother can be prevented if:
- The sensitizing event is known
- The significance of the event is realized
- The event is reported by the woman
- The practitioner acts on the knowledge
- Anti-D immunoglobulin is administered within 72 hours of the event
- Prophylactic anti-D is administered during pregnancy

will be formed. If this happens again, the body is already armed to fight the invasion of a foreign factor and haemolysis occurs. Consider a rhesus-negative woman carrying a rhesus-positive baby. If some of the baby's blood transfers across the placenta into her bloodstream, after approximately 72 hours she will develop rhesus antibodies. On this occasion there is little consequence; however, if the woman were to become pregnant again with a rhesus-positive baby, antibodies would already be present and able to cross the placenta, causing haemolysis of the fetal red blood cells (erythrocytes). The potential for harm depends on the degree of haemolysis. The developing baby may become anaemic through the development of this condition known as *haemolytic disease of the newborn (HDN)*. This is a potentially fatal condition: the fetus may develop heart failure, hydrops fetalis, or if born alive, severe jaundice. Rhesus-negative women should have their rhesus antibody status checked in early pregnancy and again at 28 weeks' gestation. For a summary of how the development of rhesus antibodies can be prevented, see Box 7.1.

Activity

Situations that increase the likelihood of blood from the fetus entering the maternal bloodstream are known as *sensitizing events*. Identify five such events.

Anti-D

If a sensitizing event is known, reported and confirmed within 72 hours, an intramuscular injection of anti-D immunoglobulin can be given to the woman to prevent her from making antibodies in response to the feto-maternal haemorrhage (FMH). Such an event can be confirmed and quantified by the Kleihauer test or the more accurate flow cytometry. This is needed to ensure that the dose given is sufficient to remove the fetal cells from circulation. Estimation of FMH is not required if the fetus is less than 20 weeks or if the fetus is known to be Rh-D negative (British Committee for Standards in Haematology 2009).

The administration of anti-D after sensitizing events was introduced in 1969. Anti-D is administered to rhesus-negative women who give birth to a rhesus-positive baby to prevent iso-immunization causing HDN in a subsequent pregnancy. This process has been very successful, and now the most vulnerable time for iso-immunization is feto-maternal transfusion in pregnancy where there has been no obvious sensitizing event. In 2002 therefore it was recommended that anti-D should be administered to all non-sensitized rhesus-negative pregnant women at 28 weeks' and 34 weeks' gestation to prevent sensitization: routine antenatal anti-D prophylaxis (RAADP) (NICE 2002). NICE (2008, 2017) continues to recommend the administration of prophylactic anti-D for rhesus-negative women; this can be given as a single dose at 28 weeks or in two doses at 28 and 34 weeks (Qureshi et al 2014).

However, RAADP implementation means that over 40,000 women each year in the UK are receiving anti-D unnecessarily because the baby's blood group is also Rh-D negative and a sensitizing event would not lead to iso-immunization. NICE now recommends that non-invasive prenatal testing is offered antenatally to Rh-D–negative women to ascertain the fetal blood group and therefore inform whether or not anti-D prophylaxis is indicated (NICE 2016). There is evidence that women welcome this opportunity, but they need appropriate information to enable them to understand the concept (Oxenford et al 2013). It is important that the 28-week sample for blood group and antibody screen is taken before the first routine prophylactic anti-D immunoglobulin (anti-D Ig) injection being given (Qureshi et al 2014).

There is a small but potential risk of anaphylaxis after administration. Also, live vaccines should not be administered within 3 months of administration of anti-D, as it will render them inactive (Jordan 2010). Anti-D can be given at the same time as the measles, mumps and rubella vaccine (MMR) using separate syringes and contralateral limbs in the postnatal period (BNF (2018)). Women who are already sensitized should not receive anti-D.

Activity

Find out how RAADP is being implemented where you work. If midwives routinely offer anti-D to non-sensitized rhesus-negative women, find out where it is administered during pregnancy and by whom. Make sure you can recognize the signs of anaphylaxis.

Red cell alloantibodies

There is also the potential for any women to make antibodies in response to exposure to foreign blood, either after sensitization from paternal red cell antigens in a previous pregnancy or through a previous blood transfusion (Joint United Kingdom Blood Transfusion and Tissue Transplantation Services Professional Advisory Committee (JPAC) 2017). Antibody screening should therefore be performed on all samples used for antenatal and pre-transfusion testing (JPAC 2017). This applies to all women irrespective of their rhesus status and should be performed in early pregnancy and again at 28 weeks' gestation (NICE 2008, 2017). Such testing enables the presence of antibodies to be picked up and then the identification of the specific antibody where appropriate. This process is important because some antibodies are more clinically significant than others: anti-D, anti-C and anti-Kell are all capable of causing severe HDN (JPAC 2017). When a woman of blood group O with immunoglobulin anti-A and anti-B is pregnant with a baby of blood group A or B, known as *ABO incompatibility*, there is the potential for HDN to develop. When a clinically significant red cell antibody is identified, the woman should be offered further investigation at a specialist centre (NICE 2008, 2017). Where one of these antibodies is identified, it is useful to have access to test the blood of the baby's father, although in some cases this may be difficult to obtain.

Activity

Consider the blood tests in Table 7.1. Find out what forms and bottles are used for each test and which laboratory each one is sent to.

Rubella antibodies

The screening programme for rubella antibodies in pregnancy has ceased as of April 2016, as it no longer meets the criteria for the UK National Screening Committee. Screening does not prevent the fetus from being exposed to the infection; of the 12 cases of congenital rubella reported between 2005 and 2015, none of these would have been averted through antenatal screening (Public Health England 2016).

Antibodies to rubella (German measles) develop either as a result of natural exposure to the infection or through immunization. All children in the UK are offered MMR at 1 year and again at 3 years, 4 months, and therefore the prevalence of measles in the UK is low. However, primary rubella infection is associated with the development of serious fetal abnormalities, including deafness, heart defects and encephalopathy. Hull and Johnston (1993) state that 85% of babies exposed to the infection in the first 8 weeks of pregnancy will have congenital abnormality. Women exposed to others with a rubella-type rash, or indeed if they themselves develop such a rash, should seek medical advice, unless known to be rubella immune.

It is recommended that women are immunized postnatally if they are known not to have been vaccinated. It is recommended that women avoid pregnancy for at least a month after immunization due to the theoretical concern that the live vaccine may be lead to fetal infection (NICE 2006, 2015; British National Formulary (BNF) 2017).

Syphilis (VDRL)

Women have been routinely tested for syphilis at the booking appointment for many years, and its incidence in Britain is now rare; 1 in 650 in 2011 had a positive screen, although 23% were false-positive results (Kingston et al 2016). Untreated syphilis may result in prematurity, perinatal death, congenital lesions and deformities; however, it can be treated effectively with penicillin, and its detection and treatment can prevent the baby from being born with congenital syphilis.

Human immunodeficiency virus (HIV)

HIV weakens the immune system and if left untreated can lead to the development of acquired immunodeficiency syndrome (AIDS) and ultimately death. All women who attend for antenatal care in the UK are offered screening for HIV with the aim of early treatment to prevent HIV transmission to the fetus or to the baby during birth or breastfeeding. A positive result affects not only the woman and her unborn baby, but also her partner, family and friends. Women who test positive for HIV should therefore be managed by a multi-professional team with a named midwife to coordinate appropriate treatment, monitoring and care. If a woman declines HIV testing, this should be documented and offered again from 26 weeks (RCOG 2010). Because of the availability of effective antiviral therapy, the mother-to-child transmission rate is now approximately 0.5% (Public Health England 2016).

Hepatitis B virus (HBV)

Hepatitis literally means *inflammation of the liver* and is caused by a viral infection. Some individuals never show signs of acute infection, although it is usual for some degree of fever, loss of appetite and general malaise to precede jaundice. For others the acute infection is severe and potentially fatal. After infection, symptoms may last for several weeks, and relapse may also occur. Individuals may then become carriers of the virus. The principal mode of transmission is by exposure to blood or blood products, and a mother can pass it to her baby. If a woman's viral status is known, however, her baby can receive a course of immunization (six in the first year of life) that can help prevent the development of carrier status. It is recommended that all pregnant women be offered HBV screening, irrespective of their potential risk. NICE continues to recommend screening for HBV in all pregnancies. However, it does not support routine testing for hepatitis C, as there is currently insufficient evidence regarding the effectiveness and cost benefits (NICE 2008, 2017).

Activity

Given that HBV transmission is via body fluids, think about who you would expect to be particularly vulnerable to this infection. Are there circumstances in which a woman should be re-tested in pregnancy for this and other infections? Describe what jaundice is. Find out what is meant by *icterus*.

Fetal abnormality screening

See Chapter 8 for details of the UK screening programme for fetal abnormality.

REFLECTION ON THE TRIGGER SCENARIO

Look back on the trigger scenario.

Joanna is now 30 weeks pregnant. She has been feeling particularly tired, and her mum suggested that she might be anaemic. Louis is rather insulted, as he prides himself on buying the best fresh ingredients from the local market; they love cooking and eat plenty of fruits and vegetables. Joanna had a full blood count taken by the community midwife who came to the flat to do her booking history.

Now that you are familiar with the schedule of blood tests in pregnancy, you should have insight into how the scenario relates to the evidence about detecting iron-deficiency anaemia. The jigsaw model will now be used to explore the trigger scenario in more depth.

Effective communication

It is essential that midwives communicate effectively with women to ensure that they can provide informed consent for the blood tests on offer. A robust and clear system of communicating blood results is also key to effective care in pregnancy. Questions that arise from the scenario might include the following: Did the midwife inform Joanna how she would let her know if she was anaemic? Who did the results go to? Is there an agreed pathway for informing and treating anaemic women? What additional information is given to women about the prevention and treatment of anaemia? What are the side effects of iron therapy? Was the result recorded in Joanna's notes at a subsequent antenatal appointment?

Woman-centred care

All women need to feel that they understand the implications of the tests on offer if they are to participate fully in their care. They need to feel able to ask questions about how a particular test might be relevant to their individual situation. Questions that arise from the scenario might include the following: Were particular tests highlighted as being particularly relevant to Joanna? Did she feel that the tests were all routine and that she had no say in whether or not she wanted them? Did Joanna feel that her results would be conveyed to her, whether or not any action was required after the results?

Using best evidence

Routinely performing blood tests on pregnant women has significant resources implications, not only in terms of financial cost but also in terms of the midwife's time. It is important therefore that unnecessary tests are not performed and that those that are routine are based on best evidence. Questions that arise from the scenario might include the following: What processes are followed when the NICE writes a new guideline or reviews its previous guidance? How is that information made available to professionals? Who disseminates this information where you work? What do NICE guidelines say about testing for and treating anaemia in pregnancy?

Professional and legal issues

Taking blood from women during pregnancy has many professional and legal implications. It is essential that midwives keep up to date with current practice and new local and national guidance. The rationale behind the various tests that midwives take is not always made explicit. Questions that arise from the scenario might include the following: Do you feel able to counsel a woman who requires a full blood count during pregnancy? Do you always inform women about the implications of an abnormal result? What does the NMC say about keeping your skills and knowledge up to date? Where do you document the results of blood tests taken?

Team working

Many professionals are involved in the care of pregnant women. Midwives rely on the development and maintenance of effective working relationships with all those who input into their care. Questions that arise from the scenario might include the following: How many professionals are involved in taking blood, undertaking the analysis, reporting the result and taking any required action based on the findings? Who else is able to take blood where you work? Whose responsibility is it to find out the results of a blood test taken by you? Does the woman have any responsibility?

Clinical dexterity

Taking blood requires considerable clinical dexterity, not only to handle the equipment, but also to find the most appropriate vein for venepuncture and disposing of the contaminated sharps. Questions that arise from the scenario might include the following: How did you learn to take blood? Do you follow trust guidance and always wear gloves when taking blood from women? Have you picked up any helpful tips by watching other professionals take blood? What are the challenges of taking blood in a woman's home?

Models of care

When blood is taken from a woman, it is important that it makes its way to the laboratory without delay. Different models of care require specific systems to be in place to ensure that blood arrives safely in the laboratory. Questions that arise from the scenario might include the following: How does blood taken in the hospital get from the ward or clinic to the laboratory? What are the collection times, or is there an automated chute system? If blood is taken in the community, how does it get from the woman's home to the laboratory? Is this system safe and effective?

Safe environment

Taking blood from a woman poses potential risks to anyone coming into that environment. For the woman, the risks include infection, haematoma and incorrect identification. Questions that arise from the scenario might include the following: Did the blood sample arrive safely in the laboratory for testing? How do you follow up the results of blood that you have taken or requested? Do you have any knowledge of the impact on the laboratory staff of receiving an inappropriately labelled blood sample? What is the procedure if this happens?

Promotes health

Every contact that a midwife has with a pregnant woman is an opportunity to enhance her general health and wellbeing. In addition to the public health benefits of counselling her regarding healthy eating to avoid or treat anaemia, treating her with kindness and respect will have a long-lasting impact on her emotional wellbeing. Questions that arise from the scenario might include the following: Did the midwife ask Joanna about her diet when she was taking blood to screen for anaemia? Did the midwife inform Joanna of sources of iron-rich food and the added benefit of consuming them in conjunction with vitamin C to enhance absorption?

Further scenarios

The following scenarios enable you to consider how specific situations influence the care the midwife provides. Use the jigsaw model to explore the issues raised in each scenario.

SCENARIO 1

Tessa is 34 weeks pregnant. She has just been to the local primary school to pick up her daughter from nursery. She overhears a group of women saying that there are two children in the school with suspected German measles. She remembers reading in one of her pregnancy books that there is a possible danger for unborn babies if their mother comes into contact with the virus.

Practice point

Most women are aware that exposure to rubella infection during pregnancy can be hazardous for the developing fetus. The danger to the fetus is highest in the first 8 weeks of gestation. However, most women in the UK are immune after the success of the childhood immunization programme.

Further questions specific to Scenario 1 include:
1. Why are pregnant women no longer tested for rubella immunity in pregnancy?

2. What action would you take if Tessa contacted you as her midwife for advice?
3. When is infection with rubella particularly hazardous for the unborn baby?
4. What are the consequences for the baby?
5. What public health measures are taken to reduce the incidence of rubella infection in the community?

SCENARIO 2

Catherine wants a home birth. She had an uneventful first labour and birth and really wants to avoid going into hospital if at all possible. Her community midwife has informed her that local policy requires her to have a haemoglobin above 105 g/L at the onset of labour. She is currently 30 weeks pregnant and her last haemoglobin was only 98 g/L.

Practice point

Anaemia in pregnancy is a widespread phenomenon that complicates the aspirations and outcomes of many pregnancies. It is responsible for an increased risk of infection, postpartum haemorrhage, general malaise and the potential need for blood transfusion. When the midwife takes blood, for whatever reason, she must ensure that the result is followed up and appropriate treatment organized. She must also ensure that the woman understands why treatment is important so that she complies with it.

Further questions specific to Scenario 2 include:
1. Why does the trust have this policy?
2. What is the evidence to suggest that women with low haemoglobin levels should give birth in hospital?
3. What action can Catherine take to increase her haemoglobin in the next 10 weeks?
4. What would happen if Catherine's haemoglobin was still low at term?
5. How would you support her as her community midwife?

Conclusion

This overview of the routine blood tests offered to pregnant women has highlighted the midwife's role as the 'font of all knowledge'. However, the midwife working within a multi-professional team can access the knowledge of specialists when an abnormality or unusual result is reported. Pregnant women are exposed to a range of tests and decisions to make. As advocates for women, midwives must continue to investigate the value of additional tests and treatments as more become available.

Resources

Anaemia in Pregnancy. Joint United Kingdom Blood Transfusion and Tissue Transplantation Services Professional Advisory Committee: https://www.transfusionguidelines.org/transfusion-handbook/9-effective-transfusion-in-obstetric-practice/9-2-anaemia-and-pregnancy

British Society for Haematology: hub for healthcare professionals. http://www.b-s-h.org.uk

Food standards agency: https://www.food.gov.uk

National Institute for Health and Care Excellence (NICE): http://www.nice.org.uk/

National Library for Health: https://www.evidence.nhs.uk

National Screening Committee: https://www.gov.uk/government/groups/uk-national-screening-committee-uk-nsc

National Study of HIV in Pregnancy and Childhood: http://www.ucl.ac.uk/nshpc/

Royal College of Obstetricians and Gynaecologists. Green top guidelines. https://www.rcog.org.uk/guidelines

References

Aghamohammadi, A., Zafari, M., Tofighi, M., 2011. High maternal hemoglobin concentration in first trimester as risk factor for pregnancy induced hypertension. Caspian J. Intern. Med. 2 (1), 194–197.

Baston, H., Hall, J., 2017. Midwifery Essentials, vol 1. Basics. Elsevier, Edinburgh.

BCSH (British Committee for Standards in Haematology, Transfusion Taskforce Working Party), 2009. Guidelines for the Estimation of Fetomaternal Haemorrhage. http://www.b-s-h.org.uk/media/15705/transfusion-austin-the-estimation-of-fetomaternal-haemorrhage.pdf. (Accessed 14 October 2017).

BNF, 2017. Measles, mumps and rubella vaccine, live. https://bnf.nice.org.uk/drug/measles-mumps-and-rubella-vaccine-live.html. (Accessed 28 January 2018).

BNF, 2018. Anti-D (Rho) Immunoglobulin. https://bnf.nice.org.uk/drug/anti-d-rh0-immunoglobulin.html. (Accessed 28 January 2018).

Chamberlain, G., Morgan, M., 2002. ABC of Antenatal Care, fourth ed. BMJ Books, London.

Hull, D., Johnston, D.L., 1993. Essential Paediatrics, third ed. Churchill Livingstone, Edinburgh.

Jordan, S., 2010. Pharmacology for Midwives – The Evidence Base for Safe Practice, second ed. Palgrave, Basingstoke.

JPAC (Joint UK Blood Transfusion and Tissue Transplantation Service Professional Advisory Committee), 2017. https://www.transfusionguidelines.org/transfusion-handbook/9-effective-transfusion-in-obstetric-practice/9-5-prevention-of-haemolytic-disease-of-the-fetus-and-newborn-hdfn. (Accessed 14 October 2017).

Khalafallah, A., Dennis, A., 2012. Iron Deficiency Anaemia in Pregnancy and Postpartum: Pathophysiology and Effect of Oral versus Intravenous Iron Therapy. J. Pregnancy 2012, 630519. http://doi.org/10.1155/2012/630519.

Kingston, M., French, P., Higgins, S., 2016. UK national guidelines on the management of syphilis 2015. Int. J. STD AIDS 27 (6), 421–446.

Luckmann, J., Sorensen, K.C., 1980. Medical and Surgical Nursing: A Psychophysiologic Approach. WB Saunders, Philadelphia.

National Institute for Health and Clinical Excellence (NICE), 2002. Technology Appraisal Guidance No 41. Guidance on the use of routine antenatal anti-D prophylaxis for RhD-negative women, London, NHS.

National Institute for Health and Care Excellence (NICE), 2006. updated 2015. Postnatal care up to 8 weeks after birth. NICE CG37. https://www.nice.org.uk/guidance/cg37. (Accessed 8 October 2016).

National Institute for Health and Care Excellence (NICE), 2008. updated 2017. Antenatal care routine care for the healthy pregnant woman: Clinical guideline 62, London, National Collaborating Centre for Women's and Children's Health.

National Institute for Health and Care Excellence (NICE), 2016. High-throughput non-invasive prenatal testing for fetal RHD genotype. Diagnostics guidance [DG25]. Available at: https://www.nice.org.uk/guidance/dg25/chapter/1-Recommendations. (Accessed 14 October 2017).

Oxenford, K., Silcock, C., Hill, M., et al., 2013. Routine testing of fetal Rhesus D status in Rhesus D negative women using cell-free fetal DNA: an investigation into the preferences and information needs of women. Prenat. Diagn. 33 (7), 688–694.

Public Health England, 2016. Rubella susceptibility screening in pregnancy ends on 1 April. https://phescreening.blog.gov.uk/2016/03/31/rubella-susceptibility-screening-in-pregnancy-ends-tomorrow/. (Accessed 14 October 2017).

Qureshi, H., Massey, E., Kirwan, D., et al., 2014. BCSH guideline for the use of anti-D immunoglobulin for the prevention of haemolytic disease of the fetus and newborn. Transfus. Med. 24 (1), 8–20. doi:10.1111/tme.12091.

Rankin, J., 2017. Physiology in Childbearing with Anatomy and Related Biosciences, fourth ed. Elsevier, Edinburgh.

Royal College of Obstetricians and Gynaecologists, 2010. Management of HIV in pregnancy. Guideline 39, Online. Available at http://doctor-ru.org/main/1300/1339.pdf.

Shuttleworth, A. (Ed.), 2002. Nursing Times Diagnostic Procedures. Emap Healthcare, London.

Steer, P., Alam, M.A., Wadsworth, J., et al., 1995. Relation between maternal haemoglobin concentration and birth weight in different ethnic groups. Br. Med. J. 310 (6978), 489–491.

Stephansson, O., Dickman, P.W., Johansson, A., et al., 2000. Maternal hemoglobin concentration during pregnancy and risk of stillbirth. JAMA 284 (20), 22–29.

CHAPTER 8

Antenatal screening for fetal abnormality

TRIGGER SCENARIO

Joanna is now 32 weeks pregnant. She is feeling quite well and finding that now her energy has returned; she is really enjoying being pregnant. She still proudly shows her precious scan picture to interested friends and takes the occasional glance at herself during quiet moments. Joanna has a cousin, Susan, who has Down's syndrome. Susan is a happy and loving child who has brought a lot of joy, as well as heartache, to the extended family. Although Joanna has no delusions about the hard work and continuing care that her cousin requires, she would not herself contemplate terminating a pregnancy if her baby had the condition.

Introduction

Antenatal screening for fetal abnormality is an integral part of routine antenatal care. It is often assumed that women will want to take up this service, just as they would have their urine tested or blood pressure checked. However, what has become routine practice for midwives can have far-reaching implications for women. This aspect of antenatal care requires the midwife to be particularly receptive to the cues that women give her and to respect the choices they make. This chapter focuses on some of the principles that are relevant to screening generally. Tests used for the diagnosis of congenital conditions are summarized, as women need to know what a positive screening test result might lead to.

What is screening?

The terms *screening* and *testing* are often used synonymously. However, they are distinctly different, and it is important that the midwife is able to convey this difference to women.

Activity

Think about anyone you know with a child who has either a physical or mental disability. Consider how caring for a disabled child affects family life. Think about the decisions you would make about screening for fetal abnormality if you were expecting a baby.

> *Screening is the process of identifying healthy people who may be at increased risk of disease or condition.*
>
> (UK National Screening Committee (UK NSC) 2013)

A population is screened to identify people who would benefit from further investigation; that is, those who have a higher risk of the condition being screened for. However, when resources are scarce or when the test itself may cause harm, screening is often limited to a sub-section of a population already deemed to be at higher risk than the rest.

When screening identifies an individual who has a 'high chance', diagnostic testing is offered to confirm or exclude the condition. Screening usually precedes diagnostic testing; however, individuals already known to be high risk because of their family or obsteteric history may opt straight for testing if it is offered. The aim of diagnostic testing is to identify if the condition is present and to offer the woman the options of continuing with her pregnancy informed by this knowledge or having a termination.

False positive and negative

Screening is not diagnostic, and it is important that the midwife understands what is meant by a positive or negative screening result. Some results will be positive, that is, fall into an at-risk group, the range of which has previously been determined. However, not all of the cases that fall into that group will have the condition, and they are termed *false positives*, a result that indicates there is a problem when there is not one.

Some results will be negative; that is, they fall outside of the previously determined at-risk range. However, not all of these cases will be free of the condition being screened for, and these are termed *false negatives*, a result that indicates there is not a problem when there is.

These are important considerations, particularly where positive screening may lead to invasive testing to confirm the presence or absence of the condition. An ideal screening test would be sufficiently sensitive to detect a high proportion of those at risk without subjecting a large number of people to unnecessary diagnostic testing.

Criteria for a screening test

The screening test should meet the following criteria stated by Public Health England (PHE 2015):

1. There should be a simple, safe, precise and validated screening test.
2. The distribution of test values in the target population should be known and a suitable cut-off level defined and agreed.
3. The test, from sample collection to result delivery, should be acceptable to the population.

4. There should be an agreed policy on the further diagnostic investigation of individuals with a positive test result and the choices available to those people.

Following wide consultation, standards have been developed and agreed by the UK NSC (2015), the body responsible for setting screening policy, that reflect both generic issues related to antenatal screening and those specific to the conditions under examination, namely Down's (trisomy 21/T21), Edwards' (trisomy 18/T18) and Patau's (trisomy 13/T13) syndromes or a number of fetal anomalies (structural abnormalities of the developing fetus). Those relating to antenatal screening tests include policy arrangements, clinical arrangements, education and training for staff, information and support for women and their partners, and audit and monitoring processes. Those specific to T21/T18/T13 screening (serum and ultrasound) comprise coverage and identifying the population, the test performance, the test turn-around time, minimizing harm, time to intervention and diagnosis. Each trust should employ a screening coordinator to facilitate the implementation of evidence-based policy and guidance (UK NSC 2011).

Activity

Make sure you are aware of how women currently receive the results of screening tests where you work. Think about who is best placed to provide an at-risk result. How would you assess a woman's capacity to consent for a screening test?

Information for women

The booking history is often the first time that women have the opportunity to discuss the issue of screening for fetal abnormality. However, the information that women receive is sometimes less than informative. Women may access information that is brief and misleading. The increase in the number of options available also adds to the confusion for prospective parents (Saller & Canick 2008), and information overload in the first trimester may detract from the important decisions around screening (Barr & Skirton 2013). The UK NSC now produces a comprehensive booklet that provides detailed information about the conditions that can be screened for and the implications of the tests (UK NSC 2017).

Lack of knowledge is not confined to pregnant women. Education and training of midwives regarding all aspects of screening is the responsibility of local screening coordinators in liaison with pre- and post-registration education providers and local trusts. However, individual midwives must also take responsibility to keep up to date with new practices and technologies (Nursing and Midwifery Council (NMC) 2015). There is a plethora of resources to support midwives in this challenging aspect of their role (PHE 2017).

The midwife must be aware that the choices women and their partners make about antenatal screening for fetal abnormality are not solely based on the information they receive in pregnancy. They may have had long-standing views after the experiences of their family and friends. Religious and cultural values will also affect the course that women take. Knowing that they would never terminate a pregnancy, for whatever reason, will prevent some women from having a screening test. Other women may be against termination but feel that they want to know if their baby has an increased risk of having a condition. Some women will feel strongly that they would want their baby, whatever problems it had. Others might feel that it is wrong to birth a baby that might have a reduced quality of life. That individuals come to a parent partnership with potentially different views also means that they need to find a stance from which they both feel comfortable, and this may take time. Other issues shown to have a positive correlation with accepting screening include 'having consanguineous marriage, a history of spontaneous abortion, a child with genetic disorder, multiparity or a longer marriage duration' (Seven et al 2017:1869).

Midwives must also be aware of the impact that their body language has on their interactions with women and demonstrate to each woman that they are listening (Baston & Hall 2017). Stapelton et al (2002) report how women often respond to midwives' apparent busyness by withholding questions and that midwives often mistake a woman's silence for lack of interest. Midwives need to make an effort to establish on what basis a woman is making a choice to ensure that she is making a decision based on understanding. The midwife has an important role in presenting balanced, relevant information in an understandable manner (Barr & Skirton 2013).

In summary

Before agreeing to have a screening test, the woman and her partner need to know:

+ What the condition involves and the implications for long-term health
+ That the test is not compulsory
+ That the midwife will support the woman, whatever choice she makes
+ What the test is for and that it is only designed to screen for a particular syndrome
+ That it is not a diagnostic test and will only give an indication of individual risk

- What the false-positive and false-negative rate is and what this means
- That they might be offered further tests if they are found to be 'high risk'
- That the diagnosis can only be made after an invasive procedure which has a 1% risk of miscarriage
- How results will be given

Understanding risk

Agreed standards for antenatal screening state that 'the cut-off level used to define the population at increased risk of an affected pregnancy must be 1 in 150 at term' (PHE 2017). The booklet available for women talks in terms of 'chance' rather than 'risk' and describes a result of more than 1 in 150 as 'lower chance' and from 1 in 2 to 1 in 150 as 'higher chance': 95% of screening results will be lower chance and 5% higher chance.

Women also need to understand that a lower chance does not mean there is no chance of having an affected baby and a higher chance does not mean they would definitely have an affected baby. A low chance result should be given by 2 weeks of the test and a high chance result within 3 working days (PHE 2017).

Activity

Describe the physical and facial characteristics of babies born with trisomy 21, trisomy 18 and trisomy 13. Consider what structural abnormalities might be identified via ultrasound scan associated with these conditions.

The fetal anomaly screening programme (FASP)

The UK NSC set the policy, and FASP is responsible for its implementation. There aims to be equal access for all women to high-quality screening care that includes access to information and freedom of choice. Women can opt not to have the pregnancy screened, and this should be respected. FASP includes three genetic conditions, and women can opt to be screened for none, one (T21), two (T18/T13) or all (T21, T18/T13).

Down's syndrome (T21)

The incidence of Down's syndrome is 1 in 1000 births in the general population and is the result of an extra chromosome 21 (PHE 2017). The chance of having an affected baby increases with maternal age, although approximately 70% of cases of Down's syndrome occur with women under the age of 36 years (Mutton et al 1998). Children born with Down's syndrome will have learning disabilities, but these vary from severe to

Table 8.1: Forms of Edwards' syndrome (T18)

Form	Chromosome copies	Prognosis
Complete trisomy 18	Every cell in the body has three copies of chromosome 18.	Fatal condition. Babies will have complex disabilities and usually die before birth or soon after.
Mosaic trisomy 18	Some cells have the usual two copies of chromosome 18 and some have three copies.	If born alive, may live beyond a year but this is rare. Complex physical and learning difficulties.
Partial trisomy 18	There is an extra part of some of chromosome 18 in all the body's cells.	If born alive, may live beyond a year but this is rare. Complex physical and learning difficulties.

being able to attend mainstream school with extra support. Although they are more likely to have heart anomalies and difficulties with sight and hearing, many grow up to have a good quality of life and to live independently with support.

Edwards' syndrome (T18)

This is a fatal condition, and most babies who have the condition die before birth or soon afterwards. Its incidence is about 3 in 10,000 births (PHE 2017). There are three forms of the condition, depending on the distribution of extra copies or parts of chromosome 18 (see Table 8.1). Because this is a fatal condition, women who have a fetus diagnosed with Edwards' syndrome are offered feticide or the option of palliative care.

Patau's syndrome (T13)

As with Edwards' syndrome, babies with Patau's syndrome usually die before they are born or soon afterwards, and therefore parents would be offered termination of the pregnancy or supportive palliative care. These babies have an extra chromosome 13, and the incidence in the general population is about 2 in 10,000 births (PHE 2017). Babies born with this condition often have heart, kidney and brain abnormalities; malformations of ears, eyes and palate; and are unable to stand.

Activity

Consider the criteria for screening tests used by the National Screening Committee (NSC). Decide how far the current screening programme in your locality fulfils these criteria.

Table 8.2: Markers for T21/T13/T18 syndromes screening in pregnancy

When	Name	Markers
10 weeks–13 weeks+ 6 days	Combined test	Serum hCG Serum PAPP-A Ultrasound nuchal translucency
14 weeks–20 weeks	Double	Serum hCG Serum uE3
14 weeks–20 weeks	Triple	Serum hCG Serum uE3 Serum AFP
14 weeks–20 weeks	Quadruple	Serum hCG Serum uE3 Serum AFP Serum inhibin A

AFP, Alpha feto protein; hCG, beta-human chorionic gonadotrophin; PAPP-A, Pregnancy-associated plasma protein A; uE3, unconjugated oestriol

The combined test

The woman must have had detailed information on which to base her decision to consent to the test. If she accepts this first trimester screening (between 10 and 13+6 days gestation), she should have both components performed: serum biochemistry and nuchal translucency (NT) measurement by ultrasound. A maternal venous blood sample is taken by the midwife or phlebotomist. Measurement of markers (Table 8.2) detected in maternal serum is combined with maternal and gestational age in the calculation of individual risk. Adjustments are made according to maternal weight, so this must be recorded when the test is taken. It has been established that other maternal characteristics, such as ethnic origin, conception via in vitro fertilization and smoking, can influence the levels of serum markers in the blood (Kagan et al 2008).

If the pregnancy is further advanced or the NT cannot be measured, women should be offered either the 'triple' or 'quadruple' serum screening test, between 14 weeks 0 days and 20 weeks 0 days.

Ultrasound screening

The use of scanning in the UK is accepted practice. Not only do women expect to have at least two scans during their pregnancy, but they also expect that they will be able to purchase a picture of their unborn baby and in some cases be informed of the baby's sex. Seeing the baby on screen helps make the pregnancy seem more real for both the woman and her partner. Having a scan in pregnancy is often anticipated as a positive experience, and although it is important not to detract from this opportunity to 'see' their developing baby, women need to be informed that the purpose is to look for abnormalities. They should also know that although this scan is available to all women, that does not mean they are obliged to have it. The sensitivity of the scan performed will depend on the resolution of the equipment used, the skill of the ultrasonographer, the gestation and the position of the baby.

The dating scan

From a clinical point of view, the use of routine scanning to date the pregnancy has been justified over the use of last menstrual period because it has been shown to reduce the number of inductions for post-maturity (Hogberg & Larsson 1997). Estimation of gestational age by ultrasound rather than on menstrual history also improves the accuracy of serum screening tests (Brennand & Cameron 2001). National guidance recommends that women have a dating scan after 10 weeks (NICE 2008, 2017). The NT thickness is measured at this scan because the fluid that collects behind the neck of the fetus is increased in those who have an abnormality.

The mid-pregnancy scan

This scan looks for physical abnormalities in the fetus and includes examination of the brain, heart, kidneys, abdomen, spine, skeleton and face. It will identify major structural abnormalities, such as 9 out of 10 cases of spina bifida, but some, such as heart defects, may be difficult to detect, and others may not develop until later in the pregnancy. As a medical examination, women should know what to expect and give their consent.

Activity

What is nuchal translucency (NT)? How is it measured, and what is its relevance to screening? How would you describe NT to women in your care? What specific observations are made during the 18- to 21-week scan?

Haemoglobinopathies

Haemoglobin is a protein that is found in the red blood cells of the blood that carries oxygen around the body. A haemoglobinopathy is a genetic (therefore inherited) abnormality of haemoglobin; in the United Kingdom the most common are sickle cell anaemia and thalassaemia.

Sickle cell anaemia

This is a recessive genetic disorder; therefore both parents need to be carriers (have sickle cell trait) for a person to inherit sickle cell disease. In this condition the affected person has abnormal red blood cells because of an abnormality of the haemoglobin – a form known as *Hb-S*. During situations where oxygen is scarce, for example, during exercise or stress, the red blood cells become 'banana' shaped and clump together. This can lead to small blood vessels becoming blocked, which deprives the area of oxygen and causes severe pain; this is known as a *sickle cell crisis*.

Thalassaemia

Thalassaemia is a term used to describe recessive genetic disorders that result in a reduction in the amount of haemoglobin produced by the body. There are two types of thalassaemia, alpha and beta, depending on the type of globin chains that are too few in number.

In alpha thalassaemia, carriers often have anaemia, with reduced mean corpuscular haemoglobin and mean corpuscular volume due to the production of insufficient alpha globin chains. If no alpha globin is produced because of no functioning alpha genes, this is incompatible with life (alpha thalassaemia major).

In beta thalassaemia, if one affected gene is inherited, the person has 3.5% abnormal haemoglobin and is a carrier but does not have the disease. However, if beta thalassaemia major is inherited, the affected person will have severe anaemia leading to death if untreated. Individuals can survive if they have regular blood transfusions or a successful bone marrow transplant. Complications of the disease include organ failure, skeletal deformity and reduced life expectancy.

Screening for haemoglobinopathies

All pregnant women should be screened for haemoglobinopathy in early pregnancy (NICE 2008, 2017). In low-prevalence areas (fetal prevalence 1.5 affected cases per 10,000 pregnancies or fewer), women should be asked to complete the Family Origin Questionnaire (FOQ) to identify if they have an increased risk. In high-prevalence areas (fetal prevalence above 1.5 affected cases per 10,000 pregnancies) or where women in low-prevalence areas are identified as being at risk through the FOQ, women should be offered laboratory screening (high-performance liquid chromatography). If the woman is subsequently identified as a carrier of either sickle cell disease or thalassaemia, the father of the baby should also be offered information and counselling and possible screening (NICE 2008, 2017).

Antenatal diagnostic tests

If a woman is found to have an increased chance of having a baby with an abnormality after screening or significant family or obstetric history, she will be offered diagnostic testing.

Cytogenetic techniques

Cytogenetics is the study of chromosomes and the related disease states caused by numerical and structural chromosome abnormalities. The process of identifying the chromosomal makeup of an individual is called *karyotyping*. To obtain a diagnosis, the fetal chromosomes are examined in the laboratory. Normally, in a human cell, there are 23 pairs of chromosomes (46 in total), but there is a range of conditions where this complement is abnormal. This process of examination involves identifying the chromosomes and hence requires the fetal cells to be sufficiently grown.

Methods for examining chromosomes continue to be developed, enabling results to be obtained faster than before. For example, fluorescent in situ hybridization is a technique which involves looking at a specific chromosome rather than all of them and takes about 3 days, thus providing a comparatively quick result (Thein et al 2000).

More recently advances in DNA sequencing technologies have enabled the detection of fetal DNA fragments. This cell-free fetal DNA (cffDNA) is detectable in maternal plasma from the first trimester, and is now being used to detect fetal Rh-D status to inform the use of prophylactic anti-D in Rh-D–negative women (see Chapter 7).

There are other applications of cffDNA analysis, using the technique of real-time polymerase chain reaction to determine fetal sex, which can be used to avoid invasive testing for sex-specific conditions, once the fetal sex is determined (Devaney et al 2011). Such non-invasive prenatal testing can potentially determine the fetal genotype, reducing the need for invasive testing in the future (Royal College of Obstetricians and Gynaecologists (RCOG) 2014, 2015). Although gaining in precision, cffDNA testing is of limited availability, depending on the facilities and skills available in the local laboratory.

> **Activity**
>
> What is maternal plasma massively parallel sequencing (MPS)? What factors make this technique less reliable? What does the International Society for Prenatal Diagnosis recommend? What is the role of fetal radiology and fetoscopy?

Cell karyotyping

Procedures for obtaining fetal cells for karyotyping include amniocentesis, chorionic villus sampling and cordocentesis.

Before agreeing to diagnostic testing, the woman and her partner need to know:

- What the test involves
- That it can detect other chromosomal abnormalities
- That there is a risk of miscarriage or infection
- That the result may take up to 3 weeks
- That occasionally the fetal cells do not grow and a result cannot be given
- How results will be given
- That they would be offered termination of the pregnancy if Down's syndrome was diagnosed

Amniocentesis

This procedure is usually carried out from 15 weeks of pregnancy. It involves removal of about 10 to 20 ml of amniotic fluid from around the fetus and is performed using ultrasound guidance. Fetal cells are cultured, and this can take up to 3 weeks or more. Sometimes, but rarely, the cells fail to grow. There is an associated miscarriage rate of approximately 1%, and there is also a small risk of infection, bleeding and premature rupture of the fetal membranes.

Chorionic villus sampling

This procedure involves removal of a sample of villi from the chorion frondosum, either transcervically or through the abdomen, and has the advantage of being performed during the first trimester of pregnancy, usually between 11 and 13 weeks. Provisional results are usually available within 1 week, as fetal cells do not need to be cultured. There is an associated 2% to 3% miscarriage rate, but because it is performed during the first trimester, it is difficult to determine which miscarriages might have occurred naturally.

Cordocentesis

Percutaneous umbilical blood sampling, or cordocentesis, involves inserting a needle through the woman's abdomen directly into the umbilical artery or vein to take a sample of fetal blood. It is performed under ultrasound guidance and carries the risks associated with amniocentesis. It is not normally attempted before 18 weeks' gestation and is not routinely used for diagnostic purposes in the UK.

REFLECTION ON THE TRIGGER SCENARIO

Look back on the trigger scenario.

Joanna is now 32 weeks pregnant. She is feeling quite well and finding that now her energy has returned; she is really enjoying being pregnant.

She still proudly shows her precious scan picture to interested friends and takes the occasional glance at herself during quiet moments. Joanna has a cousin, Susan, who has Down's syndrome. Susan is a happy and loving child who has brought a lot of joy, as well as heartache, to the extended family. Although Joanna has no delusions about the hard work and continuing care that her cousin requires, she would not herself contemplate terminating a pregnancy if her baby had the condition.

Now that you are familiar with the issues regarding antenatal screening for fetal abnormality, you should have insight into how the scenario relates to current midwifery practice. The jigsaw model will now be used to explore the trigger scenario in more depth.

Effective communication

Communication between the midwife and expectant parents is paramount if the midwife is to ensure that they understand the implications of undergoing antenatal screening for fetal abnormality. Questions that arise from the scenario might include the following: What information did Joanna receive about antenatal screening for fetal abnormality? When did she receive it and in what format? Did Joanna share the information with her partner, Louis? Did she understand the information she received? Did she have the opportunity to ask the midwife for clarification about aspects of the screening on offer?

Woman-centred care

Any screening programme, whether locally developed or following national guidelines, must ultimately be tailored to the individual needs of the family expecting the baby. Everyone comes to pregnancy with their own catalogue of hopes and fears, and these need to be acknowledged if the pregnancy is to be a positive experience. Questions that arise from the scenario might include the following: Did the midwife ask Joanna if she had thought about the implications of having a baby with Down's syndrome? Did Joanna talk about her cousin Susan when she discussed screening tests with the midwife? Was there enough time for Joanna to voice her own particular view about having a baby with Down's syndrome? Did Joanna feel any pressure to have a serum screening test?

Using best evidence

When making a potentially life-and-death decision, the woman should feel that it has been based on the best available evidence. She should feel that the midwife is giving her information based on a sound understanding of the current knowledge base. Questions that arise from the scenario might include the following: What resources can the midwife provide for women who are making decisions about antenatal screening? Is there an audit of the process and the outcome of antenatal screening for fetal abnormality? What action has been taken recently to enhance the antenatal screening service that Joanna has accessed?

Professional and legal issues

Before undergoing screening for fetal abnormality, it is essential that women are able to give informed consent. This means that information has to be presented in such a way that it is meaningful and makes sense to both the woman and her partner. Questions that arise from the scenario might include the following: What aspects of the NMC Code (NMC 2015) are particularly pertinent to gaining informed consent from a woman? What action should be taken by the midwife if a woman declines screening? What is the law around termination of pregnancy for fetal abnormality? Under what circumstances can a midwife perform ultrasonography?

Team working

Screening for fetal abnormality involves a range of professionals, each with a valuable and essential role to take, from venepuncture to conveying the result. There is a need for a robust care pathway to ensure that each member of the team takes responsibility for their particular role. Questions that arise from the scenario might include the following: Who did Joanna meet in relation to considering antenatal screening for fetal abnormality? How would the fact that Joanna declined the test be viewed by the antenatal screening coordinator? Did Joanna's partner agree with the stance Joanna has taken? How might his attitude have influenced her decision?

Clinical dexterity

The midwife involved in screening for fetal abnormality needs to have developed dexterity in handling a range of clinical scenarios. She needs to be able to give impartial information to women considering screening and also be able to inform some women that their result has placed them at high risk of having an affected baby. Questions that arise from the scenario might include the following: What do women expect from their midwife throughout the screening process? Are all midwives adept at breaking bad news? What was Joanna's midwife's reaction to her declining screening?

Models of care

Women access maternity services through a variety of systems. Some go straight to their general practitioner (GP) when they discover they are pregnant, and others access maternity services by going directly to a midwife. Questions that arise from the scenario might include the following: At what point was Joanna given information to help her make the right choice for her individual circumstances? Did she think about these issues before she had even become pregnant? What facts might make a woman change her mind? Does the profession of the person who counsels her regarding the tests available make a difference to her decision?

Safe environment

When a woman decides to have or to decline a screening test, she needs to feel secure in the decision she has made. She needs to have gone through a process whereby the decision is as clear and unambiguous as possible, having had the opportunity to explore the implications thoroughly. Questions that arise from the scenario might include the following: What organizational factors could compromise the safety of a woman's decision regarding antenatal screening? What emotional, social and cultural factors might impact on Joanna's decision to decline screening? What support will Joanna have if she births a baby with Down's syndrome?

Promotes health

The midwife has a key role to play in facilitating positive physical and emotional wellbeing for the woman and her family throughout the childbirth continuum. The midwife must therefore respect the woman's autonomy and agency to make decisions that are right for her. Questions that arise from the scenario might include the following: How can the midwife demonstrate her respect for Joanna and support her in her choices? What resources can the midwife provide for women who are contemplating pregnancy and wanting to adopt a healthy lifestyle in preparation?

Further scenarios

The following scenarios enable you to consider how specific situations influence the care the midwife provides. Use the jigsaw model to explore the issues raised in the scenario.

SCENARIO 1

Claire is 6 weeks pregnant with her first baby. She has just been to see her GP, who asked her if she was taking folic acid. When Claire said that she was not, the GP told her to start taking it, as it might reduce her chances of having a baby with spina bifida.

Practice point

Whilst the potential benefits of taking folic acid preconceptually are well understood by maternity care professionals, not all women are aware of this important public health message. Also, as many pregnancies are not planned, there may be delay in starting folic acid for those women who were aware of this advice but did not intend to become pregnant.

Further questions specific to Scenario 1 include:
1. When does the neural tube develop and close?
2. What is the recommended dose of folic acid in pregnancy?
3. Which women are at increased risk of having a baby with a neural tube defect?
4. Which foods are naturally rich in folic acid?
5. Which foods are fortified with folic acid?
6. What are the physical sequelae for a child with spina bifida?

SCENARIO 2

Gemma was born in the United Kingdom, and both her parents are African Caribbean. Two months ago she went on holiday with her friends to Morocco and met a local man, Theo, whom she began dating. They were inseparable all holiday, and she has kept in touch with him through email and texting ever since. Last week she was delighted to find out that she is pregnant with his baby.

Practice point

Some haemoglobinopathies are more prevalent in certain populations, for example, sickle cell disease. In the UK, the FOQ is a useful tool to determine whether to offer screening to a particular couple. Screening offers the opportunity to identify families with an increased chance of passing on these conditions to their children so that further genetic counselling can be provided regarding the implications for them.

Further questions specific to Scenario 2 include:
1. Which haemoglobinopathies is Gemma's baby at risk of inheriting?
2. How would this risk be verified at the booking appointment?
3. Where should Gemma be referred for expert counselling?

4. Which professionals provide genetic counselling?
5. How can Gemma involve Theo in the counselling process?

Conclusion

Antenatal screening and diagnosis for fetal abnormality is a complex issue. Midwives are required to continually update their knowledge and skills. This aspect of antenatal care presents many challenges as new programmes and technologies come into the arena, and midwives need to work closely with the multi-professional team to provide a seamless service for antenatal women.

Resources

Antenatal results and choices: Support for parents and professional. http://www .arc-uk.org/

Family origin questionnaire screening for haemoglobinopathy. https://www .gov.uk/government/publications/family-origin-questionnaire-sickle-cell-and -thalassaemia-screening

Royal College of Midwives, i-learn, Delivering unexpected news in pregnancy (professional and practice category). http://www.ilearn.rcm.org.uk

Parents' stories: personal experiences of sickle cell and thalassaemia screening. https:// phescreening.blog.gov.uk/2017/09/01/parents-stories-personal-experiences -of-sickle-cell-and-thalassaemia-screening/

Public Health England 2017 PHE Screening. We've updated the antenatal and newborn screening programmes e-learning resource. https://phescreening .blog.gov.uk/2017/01/13/weve-updated-the-antenatal-and-newborn-screening -programmes-e-learning-resource/

UK Newborn Screening Programme Centre Glossary of terms: http://www.ich .ucl.ac.uk/newborn/glossary/index.htm

References

Barr, O., Skirton, H., 2013. Informed decision making regarding antenatal screening for fetal abnormality in the United Kingdom: a qualitative study of parents and professionals. Nurs. Health Sci. 15 (3), 318–325.

Baston, H., Hall, J., 2017. Midwifery Essentials, vol 1. Basics. Elsevier, Edinburgh.

Brennand, J., Cameron, A., 2001. Current methods of screening for Down syndrome. Obstet. Gynaecol. 3 (4), 191–197.

Devaney, S.A., Palomaki, G.E., Scott, J.A., et al., 2011. Noninvasive fetal sex determination using cell-free fetal DNA: a systematic review and meta-analysis. JAMA 306 (6), 627–636.

Hogberg, U., Larsson, N., 1997. Early dating by ultrasound and perinatal outcome: a cohort study. Acta Obstet. Gynecol. Scand. 76 (10), 907–912.

Kagan, K., Wright, D., Spencer, K., et al., 2008. First-trimester screening for trisomy 21 by free beta-human chorionic gonadotrophin and pregnancy associated plasma protein-A: impact of maternal and pregnancy characteristics. Ultrasound Obstet. Gynecol. 31 (5), 493–502.

Mutton, D., Ide, R.G., Alberman, E., 1998. Trends in prenatal screening for diagnosis of Down's syndrome: England and Wales, 1987–97. Br. Med. J. 317 (7163), 922–923.

National Institute for Health and Care Excellence (NICE), 2008, updated 2017. Antenatal care: for uncomplicated pregnancies. CG62. https://www.nice.org.uk/guidance/cg62. (Accessed 28 September 2017).

Nursing and Midwifery Council, 2015. The code: professional standards of practice and behaviour for nurses and midwives. https://www.nmc.org.uk/globalassets/sitedocuments/nmc-publications/nmc-code.pdf.

Public Health England, 2015. Guidance: Criteria for appraising the viability, effectiveness and appropriateness of a screening programme. https://www.gov.uk/government/publications/evidence-review-criteria-national-screening-programmes/criteria-for-appraising-the-viability-effectiveness-and-appropriateness-of-a-screening-programme#the-test.

Public Health England, 2017. PHE Screening. We've updated the antenatal and newborn screening programmes e-learning resource. https://phescreening.blog.gov.uk/2017/01/13/weve-updated-the-antenatal-and-newborn-screening-programmes-e-learning-resource/. (Accessed 15 October 2017).

Royal College of Obstetricians and Gynaecologists, 2014, reviewed 2015. Non-invasive prenatal testing for chromosomal abnormality using maternal plasma DNA. Scientific Impact Paper No 15. https://www.rcog.org.uk/globalassets/documents/guidelines/scientific-impact-papers/sip_15_04032014.pdf. (Accessed 15 October 2017).

Saller, D., Canick, J., 2008. Current methods of prenatal screening for Down syndrome and other fetal abnormalities. Clin. Obstet. Gynecol. 51 (1), 24–36.

Seven, M., Akyüz, A., Eroglu, K., et al., 2017. Women's knowledge and use of prenatal screening tests. J. Clin. Nurs. 26 (13-14), 1869–1877. doi:10.1111/jocn.1349.

Stapelton, H., Kirkham, M., Curtis, P., et al., 2002. Silence and time in antenatal care. Br. J. Midwifery 10 (6), 393–396.

Thein, A.T., Abdel-Fattah, S.A., Kyle, P.M., Soothill, P.W., 2000. An assessment of the use of interphase FISH with chromosome specific probes as an alternative to cytogenetics in prenatal diagnosis. Prenat. Diagn. 20 (4), 275–280.

UK National Screening Committee, 2011. NHS Fetal anomaly screening programme. Failsafe processes, version 1.1. https://www.gov.uk/government/uploads/system/uploads/attachment_data/file/395144/FASP_Failsafe_processes_v1_1__2_.pdf. (Accessed 15 October 2017).

UK National Screening Committee, 2013. NHS population screening explained. https://www.gov.uk/guidance/nhs-population-screening-explained. (Accessed 14 October 2017).

UK National Screening Committee, 2015. NHS Fetal anomaly screening programme: Standards 2015-16. https://www.gov.uk/government/uploads/system/uploads/attachment_data/file/421650/FASP_Standards_April_2015_final_2_.pdf. (Accessed 15 October 2017).

UK National Screening Committee, 2017. Screening tests for you and your baby. https://www.gov.uk/government/uploads/system/uploads/attachment_data/file/674470/Screening_tests_for_you_and_your_baby_booklet.pdf.

Monitoring fetal wellbeing during routine antenatal care

TRIGGER SCENARIO

Joanna is now 36 weeks into her pregnancy and feeling well but tired. The baby seems to be most active at night when she is trying to sleep – Joanna doesn't seem to notice the movements during the day. Jo has developed some stretch marks at the top of her legs and is hoping that they will not appear on her tummy, as she likes wearing low-waisted jeans. Her partner has only heard the baby's heartbeat from a recording on Jo's phone, and is hoping to take time off work to go with her to the next antenatal appointment.

Introduction

A significant aspect of the midwife's role in the antenatal period is to monitor the health of the woman and of her unborn child. This chapter focuses on the role of the midwife in monitoring the wellbeing of the developing fetus during routine antenatal care. Because antenatal care usually takes place within the community setting in the United Kingdom, this chapter will concentrate on the antenatal examination within this arena. The skill of abdominal palpation with regard to monitoring growth, activity and the fetal heart rate will be described.

Background

Consideration for the wellbeing of the fetus should not be taken in isolation from the wellbeing of the mother, as they are both intrinsically interlinked. Pregnancy is a time of change for women and their families, and the relationship she has with her unborn baby is complex (Guedeney & Tereno 2010). Many fear that the wellbeing of their baby may have been inadvertently compromised by their social behaviour or exposure to environmental hazards. Women who conceive via assisted reproductive technology are particularly fearful of miscarriage and fetal death (Dornelles et al 2014). Part of a midwife's role is to enhance a woman's wellbeing through reassurance that her baby is growing and developing at an appropriate rate, through clinical monitoring techniques.

National guidance

The National Institute for Health and Care Excellence (NICE) guidelines for antenatal care (NICE 2008, 2017) provide direction for caring for the woman and her fetus. They outline a schedule of antenatal appointments (10 for nulliparous women and 7 for multiparous women) for women who are experiencing an uncomplicated pregnancy. However, there should be flexibility to adjust care planning dependent on her individual needs. Such personalized care, where continuity of carer is a key component, will help promote safer care that is positively appraised by women (The National Maternity Review 2016).

Professional guidance

Pre-registration midwifery standards require the student midwife to learn skills of communication in the antenatal period, as well as to 'assess and monitor women holistically' through the whole pregnancy continuum. This is carried out 'through the use of a range of assessment methods to reach valid, reliable and comprehensive conclusions'; further, student midwives need 'to carry out examinations necessary for the monitoring of the development of normal pregnancies' (Nursing and Midwifery Council (NMC) 2009).

Activity

Access the NICE antenatal guideline at https://www.nice.org.uk/guidance/cg62/chapter/1-Guidance#fetal-growth-and-wellbeing and the International Confederation of Midwives' (ICM) definition of a midwife at http://internationalmidwives.org/assets/uploads/documents/CoreDocuments/ENG%20Definition_of_the_Midwife%202017.pdf. Consider the midwife's role in monitoring the growth of the baby in relation to these standards.

Monitoring fetal wellbeing
Assessing fetal growth

During the antenatal examination, the midwife uses a range of methods to assess fetal growth, including sensitive use of discussion, palpation and measurement.

Discussion with the woman

Probably the most important gauge of fetal growth is the woman's own estimation. She is the one who is living with her growing uterus and able to note the impact of her changing shape on her daily life. She may be finding it more difficult to bend over and pick dropped items from the floor as fundal height increases. Alternatively, earlier in pregnancy she might be concerned that she has not yet needed to buy any maternity clothes. A simple question such as, 'How do you think your baby has grown since we last met?' provides an opportunity for her to voice any concerns.

Women may worry about the growth of their baby at both ends of the scale. Fear that it is growing rapidly may raise doubts about her ability to have a vaginal birth. Worry that the baby is too small may cause concern about its development and health. Concern about fetal growth can also change over time, with women worrying that they are not growing enough in early pregnancy and then too much as pregnancy advances and thoughts of the birth become more prominent.

Verbal consent to palpate the woman's abdomen should be gained at each examination. Although it will not be appropriate to launch into a full-blown explanation about what you are going to do each time you meet, if you have never met the woman before or it is the first time she has attended the clinic, she needs to know what the palpation will involve. As a midwife, you will develop your own way of asking permission to undertake procedures, but avoid the use of statements such as, 'I'm just going to …' or 'Just pop up on the couch'. Consent should not be assumed, and such language can come across as condescending. Where any language difficulties are anticipated, an interpreter should be used.

Having ensured that the woman does not have a full bladder, that she understands what you aim to do and that she agrees to it, ask her to sit on the couch. She should be asked to undo or loosen her clothing before you lower the headrest so that she can see what she is doing. The headrest should not be totally flat. Her legs should be covered with a modesty sheet and her arms by her side. The equipment required for palpation is listed in Box 9.1.

Inspection

The first observation that the midwife makes before she lays her hands on the woman is to inspect the abdomen for shape, scars, skin and size (the four S's):

Shape

The uterus of the primigravida is ovoid in shape compared with the more rounded shape of multigravida. The abdomen should be inspected for curves and dips that might give clues regarding the fetal position. If the fetus has adopted an anterior position, it may be possible to detect the curve of the fetal back. A fetus in the posterior position might give the abdomen a dip or hollow (best observed by looking at the abdomen at eye level).

Box 9.1 Equipment required for abdominal palpation

- Pinard's stethoscope
  Rationale: To locate the fetal heart
- Doppler
  Rationale: To enable the woman/partner/children to hear the fetal heart
- Aqueous jelly
  Rationale: To facilitate contact with the Doppler transducer and maternal abdomen
- Tissues
  Rationale: To remove excess jelly from the woman's abdomen
- Disposable or washable tape measure
  Rationale: To measure the symphysis–fundal height
- Modesty sheet
  Rationale: To cover the woman's legs

Scars

Abdominal scars should be noted and should correspond with the previous medical history taken at the booking visit. Women may need reassurance that a scar will not burst open, but that the skin will gradually stretch to accommodate the growing fetus.

Activity

List three indications for abdominal surgery. For each one, note down where you would expect to find the scar. Think about why it is important that scars are noted during abdominal palpation.

Skin

A line of pigmentation (linea nigra) may be noted extending centrally from the symphysis pubis to the umbilicus. The skin might appear tight and shiny if there is an excess of amniotic fluid (polyhydramnios), and further clinical signs should be considered to identify a potential case requiring referral to a medical practitioner (NMC 2015). Of considerable distress to some women is the development of stretch marks (striae gravidarum). These appear as red lines that eventually fade to silver after the birth. However, they can be itchy and cause considerable irritation, and the midwife should acknowledge the woman's discomfort, offering practical advice as well as listening to her concerns. Keeping cool and keeping the skin well moisturized and hydrated may prevent further exacerbation of this condition. Many preparations are available on the market for the 'prevention' and treatment of stretch marks; however, there is no robust evidence of their benefit (Brennan et al 2012).

> **Activity**
>
> Find out what potential fetal anomalies are associated with polyhydramnios and oligohydramnios. Make sure you know what the woman might complain of when there is excess amniotic fluid. Make yourself aware of the clinical significance of acute and/or chronic polyhydramnios.

Size

The first estimation of fetal growth is made by the midwife when she observes the abdomen. However, this is only part of the picture and one that can be entirely misleading, depending on the tone of the abdominal musculature, the amount of amniotic fluid, the accumulation of subcutaneous fat and fetal position. Further clinical assessments are required before fetal size can be more accurately judged (see the section Measurement of fundal height).

Palpation

This essential practical skill takes time to develop and, like all skills, improves with practice. The hands of a midwife become her most powerful tools, with which she can convey care as well as detect both maternal and fetal wellbeing.

Before the procedure, the woman should be encouraged to empty her bladder. She might be advised to go to the toilet when she arrives at the antenatal clinic rather than during the consultation, but her comfort should be reassessed before the palpation. If she is trying to hold on to a full bladder, her abdominal muscles may be tense and palpation uncomfortable. A full bladder can significantly affect fundal height (Engstrom et al 1989) and lead to undue concern about fetal growth.

Maintaining privacy and dignity throughout the palpation is essential. If possible, the examination couch should be arranged so that the woman's feet are away from the door and that her left-hand side (if the midwife is right-handed) is against a wall. There should be a fold-out step to enable the woman to reach the couch with ease and an adjustable headrest should be made use of. A sheet should be used to cover the woman's legs, even if she still has trousers on. This conveys the message that you understand that she is exposing her body and that you will continue to take steps to minimize this exposure.

The woman must feel safe and the focus of the midwife's attention at all times. Of course, this should be so during all points of contact between the woman and the midwife, but it is especially important when the woman is lying down and the midwife is standing up. This physical dominance must not be transferred into a superiority that prevents or spoils meaningful communication.

Estimation of gestational age

Although gestational age is invariably determined by ultrasound, the midwife uses her observation and palpation skills to compare the dates on the records with how the woman's abdomen appears, and the next part of the palpation involves estimation of gestational age and size. The midwife, usually standing with the woman's head to her left, uses her warm, clean hands to locate the uterine fundus. First, she applies the pads of the fingers of the left hand to the abdomen, just below the woman's xiphisternum. Using a gentle pressing movement, the midwife works her way down the abdomen until she feels the resistance of the fundus.

The midwife uses three landmarks when assessing gestational age by palpation: the xiphisternum, the umbilicus and the symphysis pubis. She estimates that at approximately 12 weeks of pregnancy, the fundus is palpable above the symphysis pubis. It rises approximately a centimetre each week thereafter, being between the pubis and the umbilicus at 16 weeks and at the umbilicus by about 22 to 24 weeks. By 32 weeks the fundus is midway between the umbilicus and xiphisternum. At 36 weeks the gravid uterus has reached the xiphisternum, and in subsequent weeks, as the presenting part enters the pelvis, the fundal height descends slightly ('lightening'). The overall size of the uterus must be taken into account, however, as fundal height will vary depending on the fetal lie.

Measurement of fundal height

The ability to assess fetal growth is a midwifery skill that develops with experience. Continuity of care in the community will aid the detection of babies whose growth begins to deviate from normal parameters. Fetal growth restriction is associated with poor neonatal outcome and accounts for 30.3% of UK stillbirths with unknown primary cause of death (Manktelow et al 2017).

In an attempt to employ a more 'objective' method of monitoring fetal size, physical measurement with a tape has been advocated. First the fundus is located (Fig. 9.1A). The tape is held at the fundus and extended to the symphysis pubis (from the variable to the fixed point). For a more objective measurement, it should be held so that the centimetre side is applied to the woman's abdomen and more than one measurement taken (Fig. 9.1B). This practice has been part of UK national guidance since 2003 and it remains a recommendation that symphysis fundal height is measured at each examination after 24 weeks' gestation (NICE 2008, 2017; Royal College of Obstetricians and Gynaecologists (RCOG) 2013, 2014). The

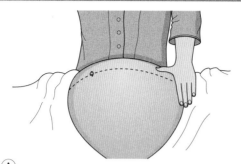

(A)   Palpate to determine fundus with two hands

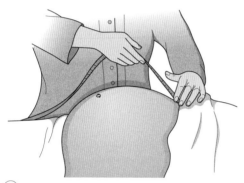

(B)   Secure tape with hand at top of fundus

Fig. 9.1 (A) Palpate the fundus. (B) Secure the tape at the top of the fundus.

measurement should be plotted on a growth chart, and any deviation as determined by local protocol must be acted upon.

Activity
Find out the local policy for measurement of fundal height in your trust. Discover what action should be taken if the fundal height plotted is a) static, b) not following the centile line but not crossing it, c) a downward trajectory crossing a centile line or d) an upward trajectory crossing a centile line.

However, this method of estimating fetal growth has been criticized for a range of reasons, including uncertainty regarding where to take the measurement from and to (Engstrom & Sittler 1993a), discrepancies between examiners (Engstrom et al 1993b) and differences in measurements due to maternal position (Engstrom et al 1993c). A Cochrane review of the controlled trials comparing symphysis–fundal height (SFH) with serial ultrasound and abdominal palpation to detect small for gestational age (SGA) fetuses concluded that there is insufficient evidence to evaluate the use of SFH measurement in pregnancy, but that a change in practice could not be recommended (Peter et al 2015).

Customized growth charts

Gardosi and Francis (1999) evaluated the use of customized charts (adjusted for maternal height, weight in early pregnancy, parity and ethnic origin) for plotting serial measurement of fundal height. They found that the use of such charts by community midwives led to an increase in the detection of SGA babies (48% in the study group compared with 29% of controls) and large for gestational age babies (46% in the study group compared with 24% of controls). Their use has not been recommended by NICE (2008, 2017) and no randomized controlled trials have compared the detection of SGA babies using customized growth charts versus population charts (Carberry et al 2014). However, their use is recommended by the RCOG (2013, 2014). The Saving Babies' Lives Care Bundle, aimed at reducing stillbirth, takes the middle ground and advocates the use of 'customised or other standardised' charts (NHSE 2016:16) and does not stipulate one over the other. However the bundle does acknowledge the value of training and standardization of measurement that goes alongside the use of customized growth charts (NHSE 2016:17). Hence many units are using customized growth charts, after staff training and implementation of specific software for the generation of bespoke charts, for each woman.

Fundal, lateral and pelvic palpation

The remainder of the palpation focuses on determining the lie, presentation and position of the fetus. The student midwife is encouraged to adopt a systematic approach to this technique and to practise translating her findings into professional language. However, she must not lose sight of the fact that the woman will need an ongoing commentary of what the midwife is feeling, and the woman should be encouraged to contribute to the detective work. Ascertaining the position and presentation of the baby is recommended at 36 weeks of pregnancy so that babies in breech presentation can be identified and women offered external cephalic version at 37 weeks (NICE 2008, 2017).

For a brief summary of abdominal palpation, see Box 9.2.

Box 9.2 Summary of abdominal palpation

- Fundal palpation

  Technique: Place both hands gently around the fundus, using the pads of closed fingers to determine contours of the fetus.

  Rationale: To determine the contents of the upper pole of the uterus. To inform pelvic palpation.

  Findings: The head feels hard and is ballotable. Note the size in relation to fundal height – breech is broader and neck is not distinguishable.

- Lateral palpation

  Technique: Imagine the uterus is half an orange and there are six segments. Facing the woman, keep left hand at the left side of the uterus (her right). Use the pads of the fingers of the right hand to work down the fundus, starting at the most lateral edge, segment 1. Keeping the left hand still, repeat from the top, but moving anteriorly to segment 2. Repeat on segment 3. Now use the right hand to steady the right side of the uterus and repeat for segments 6, 5 and 4.

  Rationale: To keep the fetus steady to enable the position of the fetal back to be identified. To use a systematic approach to locate the fetal back. To determine the position of the fetus.

  Findings: The back continues from the breech down. It is distinguishable from the irregular feel of the fetal limbs. Contours can be followed down to the shoulder and neck. Detection of the back at the far sides of uterus (segment 1–2 or 6–5) = lateral position. Location at segment 2–3 or 5–4 = anterior position. Back not easily felt but limbs felt anteriorly = posterior position.

- Pelvic palpation

  Technique: Midwife faces woman's feet and uses both hands on either side of the lower pole of the uterus, fingers together, using finger pads, not tips. May need to encourage breathing exercises or bend knees slightly. Alternative Pawlik grip uses one hand only to grasp presenting part (PP) – this is painful and not recommended. The woman is encouraged to feel PP for herself.

  Rationale: To confirm presentation and engagement. Can be uncomfortable and cause woman to 'guard' her abdomen. To involve woman in her care.

  Findings: Head feels hard and smooth, neck distinguishable. Buttocks broad and no neck felt. If fingers when placed either side of head can get round top and point inwards = not engaged. If fingers point outward around base of head, likely to be engaged.

Fetal movements

During the palpation, the midwife will involve the woman by asking her where she feels most of her movements. In combination with what she is feeling, this information will help the midwife to deduce the fetal position. In addition, she will ask the woman about the fetus's general activity and address any concerns that the woman might have. Fetal activity is used as a determinant of fetal wellbeing, as there is evidence that it may indicate placental dysfunction leading to reduction in the amount of oxygen and nutrients available to the growing fetus (O'Sullivan et al 2009). There is no evidence to suggest that routine counting of fetal movements has any beneficial outcome (Berbey et al 2001). As pregnancy advances there is less room for the baby to move, and movements therefore *feel* different; however, the baby should remain active for the whole pregnancy and, indeed, during labour. We know that when women understand the significance of fetal movements as an indicator of wellbeing, this can significantly reduce the rate of stillbirth through increased reporting (Tveit et al 2009) but we can only achieve this if we use effective methods of educating women and those who care for them (Berndl et al 2013). There is no evidence to show that increased fetal movements are of clinical significance.

Activity

Access the website 'Kicks Count' at http://www.kickscount.org.uk. Watch the video and consider what factors might lead to a woman delaying seeking professional help if her baby's movements alter. Explore what other web applications can support women to monitor their baby's activity.

The National Maternity Survey (Redshaw & Henderson 2014) asks women if they had any concerns about their baby's movements during pregnancy. Most women (53%) worried occasionally, with 14% of women worrying a great deal and 33% not worrying at all. If a woman reports reduced fetal movement (RFM), she should be managed according to her gestation and if previous episodes of reduced movements have been experienced. In addition there are a range of risk factors that make RFM more concerning, including reduced fetal growth, previous fetal demise, smoking, obesity, advanced maternal age and post-maturity. Additional medical or obstetric history would also need to be taken into account. A woman should feel that she can seek advice at any time of day or night and be greeted in such a way that she feels she could report another episode without fear of feeling she is wasting staff time (Smyth et al 2016).

Hence women should be encouraged to report a significant reduction or sudden alteration in the nature of movements from the baby's usual pattern. The Royal College of Obstetricians & Gynaecologists recommends that this important clinical sign after 28 weeks' gestation should always be taken seriously and investigated without delay (RCOG 2011).

When a pregnant woman reports a reduction in fetal movements, a cardiotocograph (not indicated if less than 28 weeks' gestation) recording fetal heart rate and fetal movements is usually performed, often in an antenatal day unit. Further investigation, such as ultrasonography for growth and liquor volume, may subsequently be requested depending on the findings. However, there is wide variation in midwives' and obstetricians' responses to women reporting reduced fetal movements, and further evidence is required in this area to inform appropriate management (Heazell et al 2008).

> **Activity**
>
> Imagine what advice you would give a woman who had not felt fetal movements by 20 weeks of pregnancy. Think about what you would say to a woman who states that her baby does not seem to be moving as much as usual.

Fetal heart rate

It is not recommended by NICE (2008, 2017) to routinely listen to the fetal heart, though a woman may find it comforting and may ask for a midwife to do so. The fetal heart can usually be detected using a Doppler as soon as the uterus is palpable above the symphysis pubis. It is often not possible to hear the fetal heart clearly through a Pinard's stethoscope before 28 weeks' gestation. Wickham (2002) provides a useful summary of the 'tips and tricks' used by midwives when listening to the fetal heart through a Pinard's stethoscope. Having identified the position of the fetal back during palpation, the midwife uses a Pinard's stethoscope (depending on gestation) to locate the fetal heart (in between the fetal shoulders) (Fig. 9.2). Clear location of the fetal heart also informs the identification of fetal position and presentation.

It is essential that the midwife develops and maintains this clinical skill to avoid difficulty in the event of Doppler battery failure, and the Pinard's stethoscope still has a valuable role where resources are limited or the woman requests limited intervention (Jauniaux & Prefumo 2016). It also enables the midwife to determine the best place to position the Doppler transducer, thus avoiding unnecessary noise distortion. The midwife can then use a Doppler so that the woman and her companion(s) can hear the fetal heartbeat. The maternal pulse should also be identified to confirm that the heart rate detected abdominally is that of the fetus. It should be auscultated for a full minute and the number of beats per minute (bpm) recorded in the woman's antenatal records. If the fetus becomes active during this time, acceleration of the fetal heart should be noted.

The fetal heart rate (FHR) varies according to gestational age. The mean FHR at 25 weeks' gestation is 150 bpm, reducing to approximately 142 bpm at term (Park et al 2001). A reassuring FHR is between 110

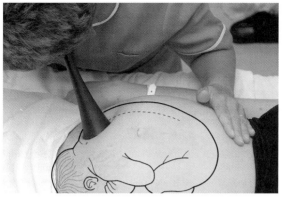

Fig. 9.2 Auscultation of the fetal heart with a Pinard's stethoscope.

and 160 bpm (NICE 2014, 2016). Any deviation from this range or irregularity detected requires referral to an obstetrician.

REFLECTION ON THE TRIGGER SCENARIO

Look back on the trigger scenario.

> Joanna is now 36 weeks into her pregnancy and feeling well but tired. The baby seems to be most active at night when she is trying to sleep – Joanna doesn't seem to notice the movements during the day. Jo has developed some stretch marks at the top of her legs and is hoping that they will not appear on her tummy, as she likes wearing low-waisted jeans. Her partner has only heard the baby's heartbeat from a recording on Jo's phone, and is hoping to take time off work to go with her to the next antenatal appointment.

Now that you are familiar with monitoring fetal wellbeing, you should have insight into how the scenario relates to the evidence about this. The jigsaw model will now be used to explore the trigger scenario in more depth.

Effective communication

During antenatal care, it is important for a midwife to use communication skills appropriately. She will need to use her skills to find out information from Joanna in order to establish the wellbeing of Joanna and her baby. Questions that arise from the scenario might include the following: Has Joanna met her midwife before? What questions may the midwife ask her to find out what has been taking place? What clues may the midwife look for to establish Jo's feelings about the wellbeing of her baby? Where will the midwife record information?

Woman-centred care

This involves a sensitive, individualized approach to care and considering the woman's needs from her perspective. In Jo's situation the midwife will consider her thoughts and needs at this time. Questions that arise from the scenario might include the following: What is concerning Jo most about the wellbeing of herself or her baby? How might the concerns about her stretch marks be addressed? How will her partner be included more in this pregnancy?

Using best evidence

In this scenario the midwife needs to consider the best evidence available to ensure fetal wellbeing is monitored effectively. Questions that arise from the scenario might include the following: Is there any evidence from Jo that the baby is not moving appropriately? Are there any maternal factors that may influence the growth of the baby? What do the stretch marks signify? What is the evidence surrounding their prevention? Which evidence supports the clinical practice of the midwife?

Professional and legal issues

Midwives should always practise within the framework of their profession and the law. In this scenario questions that need to be addressed to ensure that the woman's care fulfils statutory obligations include the following: Has the midwife been appropriately educated and mentored to give antenatal care? Is she practising according to the code of professional conduct? Are there any local, national or international guidelines relating to Jo's care? What action should the midwife take if she detects an abnormality? How would she document her care?

Team working

Though community-based midwives often work alone, they are also based within a primary health environment that involves other health professionals. It is important that they communicate with each other: each may have a particular insight into Joanna's health status. Questions that need to be addressed in this scenario are the following: Are there any indications that Jo and her baby need to be referred to another professional? If so, who will this be? Where will the midwife record information for other health professionals? How will the midwife make contact with other health professionals if required?

Clinical dexterity

In this scenario the midwife will require skill and experience to palpate Jo's abdomen, without causing undue distress or harm, and to auscultate the fetal heart, if required. Questions that could arise are the following: Has the midwife received appropriate training in the skills required? Where will this examination be carried out? How will she ensure Jo retains her dignity? What will she use to hear the fetal heart? How will she estimate fetal growth? How will she maintain her skills and pass them on to others?

Models of care

A number of models of antenatal care are currently practised by midwives in the UK. Monitoring the wellbeing of the fetus may be more ideally carried out by the same person each time, particularly in relation to monitoring fetal growth. In this situation, questions that could be raised are the following: Has this midwife met Jo before and so is able to make a judgement on changes in the growth? Would continuity of care be beneficial in this situation? Is home-based care more beneficial in this situation? Are there other professional groups involved in Jo's care who would need informing?

Safe environment

All midwifery care should be carried out in a safe environment, for the woman, her family members and the midwife. Questions that could be asked about this scenario are as follows: Are Jo and her midwife safe within the environment of care? Is any of the equipment to be used likely to put her or her baby in danger? Are there any risks to the midwife with the position in which Jo will need to be examined? How could this be altered to prevent this risk?

Promotes health

Antenatal care provides many opportunities for midwives to promote the wellbeing of the woman, her baby and her family. In this scenario questions that could be asked to ensure that the woman's care promotes physical and emotional health include the following: Are there any lifestyle issues that may be affecting Jo or the baby's health? How will the midwife find this out? What suggestions may she make to help? What suggestions may she make regarding Jo's anxieties? How may the midwife include the partner more in antenatal care?

Further scenarios

The following scenarios enable you to consider how specific situations influence the care the midwife provides. Use the jigsaw model to explore the issues raised in the scenario.

SCENARIO 1

Lisa is 39 weeks pregnant. Her husband comes home from work and says lightheartedly, 'How's nipper doing today?' Lisa sits down and suddenly realizes that she has not noticed the baby move today.

Practice point

Maintaining a normal pattern of fetal movements throughout pregnancy provides reassurance that the fetus is getting sufficient oxygen and nutrients to remain active. A sudden change in the usual pattern should alert the mother and midwife to investigate fetal health through heart rate monitoring and ultrasonography if necessary.

Further questions specific to Scenario 1 include:
1. When did Lisa last see her midwife?
2. Had there been any cause for concern at the last antenatal appointment?
3. Why might Lisa not have noticed the baby move today?
4. What should she do now?
5. What advice would you give her if you were her community midwife?

SCENARIO 2

Janice is 34 weeks pregnant. Although she has been trying really hard not to put too much weight on this time, she is already classified as 'obese'. Last time she went to clinic for a routine antenatal appointment the midwife referred her to the hospital for an ultrasound scan.

Practice point

There are some circumstances where it is difficult to use traditional methods for assessing fetal growth. Women who are obese can be difficult to measure, and as they are also at risk of faltering or accelerated fetal growth, robust assessment of the actual growth trajectory is key to assessing fetal wellbeing.

Further questions specific to Scenario 2 include:
1. Why did the midwife refer Janice for a scan?
2. What factors influence the growth of the fetus?

3. In what circumstances can it be difficult to estimate fetal growth through symphysis pubis measurement?

4. What other parameters are used to assess fetal wellbeing during routine care?

5. How should Janice's remaining care be managed?

Conclusion

Monitoring fetal wellbeing in the community setting requires the use of the midwife's skill in the clinical art of abdominal palpation. During this systematic examination the midwife not only uses her hands to confirm that the fetus is growing and active, but also uses her interpersonal skills to enable the woman to take an active part in monitoring her baby's health.

Resources

AFFIRM study (protocol) designed to test the introduction of a package of care to identify fetal compromise. http://bmjopen.bmj.com/content/7/8/e014813

Stillbirth Care Bundle: NHSE - National Health Service England 2016 Saving babies lives. A care bundle for reducing stillbirth. https://www.england.nhs.uk/wp-content/uploads/2016/03/saving-babies-lives-car-bundl.pdf

Information and videos regarding customised fetal growth charts. https://www.perinatal.org.uk/FetalGrowth/GAP/GAP.aspx

Tommy's: Reduced fetal movements resources. https://www.tommys.org/pregnancy-information/symptom-checker/reduced-fetal-movements-my-babys-movements-have-slowed-down

National Institute for Health and Care Excellence. http://www.nice.org.uk/.

Royal College of Obstetricians and Gynaecologists. http://www.rcog.org.uk/.

References

Berbey, R., Manduley, A., Gracia, V.G., 2001. Counting fetal movements as a universal test for fetal wellbeing. Int. J. Gynaecol. Obstet. 74 (3), 293–295.

Berndl, A., O'Connell, C., McLeod, N.L., 2013. Fetal movement monitoring: How are we doing as educators? J. Obstet. Gynaecol. Can. 35 (1), 22–28.

Brennan, M., Young, G., Devane, D., 2012. Topical preparations for preventing stretch marks in pregnancy. Cochrane Database Syst. Rev. (11), Art. No.: CD000066, doi:10.1002/14651858.CD000066.pub2.

Carberry, A.E., Gordon, A., Bond, D.M., et al., 2014. Customised versus population-based growth charts as a screening tool for detecting small for gestational age infants in low-risk pregnant women. Cochrane Database Syst. Rev. (5), Art. No.: CD008549, doi:10.1002/14651858.CD008549.pub3.

Dornelles, L., Maccallum, F., Lopes, R., et al., 2014. Living each week as unique: Maternal fears in assisted reproductive technology pregnancies. Midwifery 30 (3), E115–E120.

Engstrom, J.L., Ostrenga, K.G., Plass, R.V., et al., 1989. The effect of maternal bladder volume on fundal height measurements. Br. J. Obstet. Gynaecol. 96 (8), 987–991.

Engstrom, J.L., Sittler, C.P., 1993a. Fundal height measurement. Part 1 – techniques for measuring fundal height. J. Nurse Midwifery 38 (1), 5–16.

Engstrom, J.L., McFarlin, B., Sittler, C.P., 1993b. Fundal height measurement. Part 2 –intra- and interexaminer reliability of three measurement techniques. J. Nurse Midwifery 38 (1), 17–22.

Engstrom, J.L., Piscioneri, L., Low, L.K., et al., 1993c. Fundal height measurement. Part 3 – the effect of maternal position on fundal height measurements. J. Nurse Midwifery 38 (1), 23–27.

Gardosi, J., Francis, A., 1999. Controlled trial of fundal height measurement plotted on customised antenatal growth charts. Br. J. Obstet. Gynaecol. 106 (4), 309–317.

Guedeney, A., Tereno, S., 2010. Transition to parenthood. In: Tyano, S., Herrman, H., Cox, J. (Eds.), Parenthood and Mental Health: A Bridge Between Infant and Adult Psychiatry. Wiley Blackwell, UK.

Heazell, A., Green, M., Wright, C., et al., 2008. Midwives and obstetrician knowledge and management of women presenting with decreased fetal movements. Acta. Obstet. Gynecol. Scand. 87 (3), 331–339.

International Confederation of Midwives (ICM), 2017. International definition of a midwife. http://internationalmidwives.org/assets/uploads/documents/CoreDocuments/ENG%20Definition_of_the_Midwife%202017.pdf, (Accessed 16 October 2017).

Jauniaux, E., Prefumo, F., 2016. Fetal heart monitoring in labour: from pinard to artificial intelligence. BJOG 123 (6), 870.

Manktelow, B.N., Smith, L.K., Prunet, C., et al., on behalf of the MBRRACE-UK Collaboration, 2017. MBRRACE-UK Perinatal Mortality Surveillance Report, UK Perinatal Deaths for Births from January to December 2015: Summary Report. Leicester: The Infant Mortality and Morbidity Studies, Department of Health Sciences, University of Leicester.

National Institute for Health and Care Excellence (NICE), 2008, updated 2017. Antenatal care for uncomplicated pregnancies. CG62. https://www.nice.org.uk/guidance/cg62. (Accessed 28 September 2017).

National Institute for Health and Care Excellence (NICE), 2014, updated 2016. Intrapartum care: care for healthy women and babies. NICE CG190. https://www.nice.org.uk/guidance/cg190. (Accessed 16 October 2017).

National Maternity Review, 2016. Better Births. Improving outcomes of maternity services in England. Available at: https://www.england.nhs.uk/wp-content/uploads/2016/02/national-maternity-review-report.pdf.

NHSE - National Health Service England, 2016. Saving babies' lives. A care bundle for reducing stillbirth. https://www.england.nhs.uk/wp-content/uploads/2016/03/saving-babies-lives-car-bundl.pdf. (Accessed 16 October 2017).

Nursing and Midwifery Council (NMC), 2009. Standards for Pre-Registration Midwifery Education. NMC, London.

Nursing and Midwifery Council, 2015. The code: professional standards of practice and behaviour for nurses and midwives. https://www.nmc.org.uk/globalassets/sitedocuments/nmc-publications/nmc-code.pdf.

O'Sullivan, O., Stephen, G., Martindale, E., Heazell, A.E.P., 2009. Predicting poor perinatal outcome in women who present with decreased fetal movements. J. Obstet. Gynaecol. 29 (8), 705–710. doi:10.3109/01443610903229598.

Park, M.I., Hwang, J.H., Cha, K.J., et al., 2001. Computerized analysis of fetal heart rate parameters by gestational age. Int. J. Gynaecol. Obstet. 74 (2), 157–164.

Peter, R.J., Ho, J.J., Valliapan, J., Sivasangari, S., 2015. Symphysial fundal height (SFH) measurement in pregnancy for detecting abnormal fetal growth. Cochrane Database Syst. Rev. (9), Art. No.: CD008136, doi: 10.1002/14651858. CD008136.pub3.

Redshaw, M., Henderson, J., 2015. Safely Delivered: A national survey of women's experience of maternity care 2014 https://www.npeu.ox.ac.uk/downloads/files/reports/Safely%20delivered%20NMS%202014.pdf. (Accessed 17 March 2017).

Royal College of Obstetricians & Gynecologists, 2011. Reduced Fetal Movements. Green-top Guideline No. 52.

Royal College of Obstetricians & Gynecologists, 2013, 2014. The Investigation and Management of the Small-for-Gestational-Age Fetus. Green-top guideline No 31. https://www.rcog.org.uk/globalassets/documents/guidelines/gtg_31.pdf.

Smyth, R., Taylor, W., Heazell, A., et al., 2016. Women's and clinicians perspectives of presentation with reduced fetal movements: A qualitative study. BMC Pregnancy Childbirth 16 (1), 280.

Tveit, J., Saastad, E., Stray-Pedersen, B., et al., 2009. Reduction of late stillbirth with the introduction of fetal movement information and guidelines - a clinical quality improvement. BMC Pregnancy Childbirth 9, 32.

Wickham, S., 2002. Pinard wisdom. Tips and tricks from midwives (Part 1). Pract. Midwife 5 (9), 21.

Antenatal care: preparing for the birth

TRIGGER SCENARIO

Joanna is now 36 weeks into her pregnancy. She is worried about how her partner, Louis, will support her during labour. Although he has been to a couple of classes, there seems to be only one man in the group who says anything, and he has been through the process with another partner. Joanna feels that it is really important to her that Louis takes an active role during the labour. However, she worries that he may be overwhelmed and not feel comfortable with the situation.

Introduction

This chapter explores the preparations made by women and their partners as they approach the birth of their baby. Factors including antenatal expectations and preparation-for-childbirth classes will be considered. The use of birth plans as a tool to enable women and their birthing partners to discuss and clarify hopes and fears about the labour and birth will also be outlined.

Antenatal expectations

Many women will approach birth with a complex set of hopes and concerns. These will reflect many influences, including their previous experiences, the stories they have been told (Kay et al 2017) and their personality (Wiklund et al 2006). In some instances, the anticipation of the unknown generates fear of childbirth (Haines et al 2012) as highlighted in Chapter 6. The evidence is not clear regarding the most appropriate intervention to help women overcome this fear. In a small case-controlled study, women with fear of childbirth who received continuous support by a midwife in labour evaluated their experience similarly to women who did not have fear, suggesting a positive effect of the intervention (Sydsjö et al 2015). A randomized study of telephone support by midwives showed women with fear preferred a normal birth in a future pregnancy, had fewer caesarean sections and were less likely to experience flashbacks of birth (Fenwick et al 2015).

How women anticipate birth has significant sequelae for their experiences. In a large prospective study exploring women's expectations and experiences of childbirth (Green et al 2003), it was reported that women in 2000 were significantly more worried antenatally about the thought of pain in labour than were women in 1987. This increase was particularly marked for primigravid women, with 26% choosing the option 'very worried' compared with only 9% in 1987. Women in 2000 were also significantly more likely to accept obstetric intervention than their counterparts in 1987 (Green & Baston 2007). Antenatal expectations influence postnatal evaluations (van Bussel et al 2010). Midwives need to help women regain their faith in their ability to birth their babies without assistance. Further research is required to explore the most appropriate ways to enhance women's confidence and to facilitate and promote unassisted birth.

Activity

Find out what is meant by mindfulness-based childbirth education (MBAC).
  What are the perceived benefits of this approach and where is it practiced?

Preparation for birth support

Women who have high expectations have better psychological outcomes than women who have low expectations (Green et al 1998; Hildingsson 2015). Women should be encouraged to develop confidence in their abilities to cope with the challenge of labour, and this should be one of the aims of preparation-for-childbirth groups. The provision of information about the choices available, such as pain relief, will enable women to be actively involved in decisions about their care. Involvement in decision making is an important contributor to a positive birth experience, enhancing a woman's sense of control of the situation (Cook & Loomis 2012). It is highlighted by Mary Nolan (2009) that women prefer small groups with an experienced educator who will facilitate discussion and application to her needs.

In a national survey of women's experience of maternity care conducted by the National Perinatology Epidemiology Unit (NPEU) (Redshaw & Henderson 2015), 84% of first-time mothers who responded said that they had been offered antenatal groups as part of their National Health Service (NHS) England care compared with 45% of women who had already had a baby. However, not all pregnant women who are offered group participation take up the invitation; 48% of primigravid women and

91% of multigravid women did not attend. This may be for a range of reasons, groups being full, not being held at convenient times or places, not perceived as useful, etc. Further sub-group analysis revealed that younger women were more likely and black and minority ethnic women or women from a less wealthy area were less likely to be offered the groups.

Efforts have been made to provide community-based groups at different times across the week, during the day and evenings, to accommodate different demographics. Groups have also been run both to include male or female partners and to meet the needs of younger women. Groups have also been created in community centres, where there is a multidisciplinary focus. The *Better Births* report (National Maternity Review 2016) highlights projects where there are positive antenatal education activities, which includes a multidisciplinary approach.

Depending on local provision, women should be encouraged to attend groups that best meet their individual needs. Groups for women who have already had a baby, for women expecting a multiple birth or for teenagers are some examples that cater for women's specific needs rather than the 'one class fits all' approach. NICE (2008, 2017) advises that women be offered to attend participant-led antenatal groups and breastfeeding workshops.

> **Activity**
>
> Find out what childbirth preparation groups are available in your area. What gestation do they start at, who runs them and how many meetings are there in a course? Find out about Grantly Dick–Read. Who was he and what was his philosophy?

Non-NHS groups

In recent years there has been a reduction in the provision of antenatal education by midwives within many services, and the provision of non-NHS groups and activities has grown significantly. This may be in response to lack of availability, but also to the desire to have a more personal experience rather than attend a large anonymous group at the hospital. In the NPEU survey (Redshaw & Henderson 2015) it was reported that 14% of women paid for their antenatal classes. Private groups range from a luxury weekend away with like-minded couples to yoga and hypnobirthing coaching.

Physical preparation

Women can also make physical preparations for the birth. These may include attending activities designed especially for pregnant women, such as aquanatal and relaxation sessions. Preparations can also be made for an active labour by becoming familiar with and practising strategies to cope with contractions using non-pharmacological means. Women should be informed of the potential benefits of the strategies available to ensure they have realistic expectations of their effectiveness. A meta-analysis of studies highlights that upright positions and activity in the first stage of labour is beneficial as they reduce the length of labour, the potential of a caesarean birth and the need for an epidural and do not appear to cause undue harm to the woman or baby (Lawrence et al 2013). Conversely, a study comparing upright with lying positions for nulliparous women with an epidural has shown a significant increase in spontaneous vaginal birth in the lying group (The Epidural and Position Trial Collaborative Group 2017).

Women can be made to feel that the birthing room is theirs to adapt to their own needs or, alternatively, be made to feel that their requests or suggestions are too difficult to accommodate. A midwife can encourage a woman to adopt different positions or stay active during labour through positive reactions and creating an environment that enables active birth. The NPEU survey (Redshaw & Henderson 2015) reported that 82% of all women who had a vaginal birth did so on a bed, 4% on the floor and 12% in water. Two per cent used some form of birthing stool.

Student midwives can play a significant role in helping women feel that their hopes and aspirations for the birth will be acknowledged and upheld wherever possible. The fresh knowledge and enthusiasm that the student midwife brings to clinical practice can contribute to the introduction of alternative ways of working, under the close supervision of experienced midwives.

Internet-based information

Developments in Internet-based information for parents has increased dramatically with access through handheld devices and tablets. There are 'applications' (apps) that provide general or personalized information, resources from charities, resources from health departments and the NHS, resources from professional groups, international websites, Internet parenting discussion groups that provide peer support and specific sites for individual conditions or for fathers. The plethora of places where women and their families may gain information is overwhelming and can be confusing with different advice provided for the same circumstance. This is alongside the leaflets and information provided by the midwife (NICE 2008, 2017) and glossy parenting magazines purchased off the shelf.

Activity

Take some time to locate some of the information available for women for a particular topic (e.g. nutrition in pregnancy). Compare the information that is provided across all the sources. How will women know if the material provided is up to date, evidence based or relevant to them in their situation?

Women may also be active on social media, and many groups and activities use these platforms to provide information and act as discussion boards. There are questions about the nature of the information that is provided to women through all media, and television particularly, as there seems to be more portrayal of the medicalized aspects of birth as opposed to straightforward experiences (Luce et al 2016). It is suggested that there is a potential impact of increasing fear and anxiety in women (Byrom 2016), and it is important for midwives to have awareness of what women may be reading or watching via all sorts of media to be prepared to dispel these fears.

Birth plans

The ethos of maternity care in the UK is for the woman to be central to her care and for care to be individualized to her (National Maternity Review 2017; NICE 2008, 2017). *Better Births* (2017:8) states:

> *Unbiased information should be made available to all women to help them make their decisions and develop their care plan.*

Preparation-for-childbirth groups can be a valuable resource for women when it comes to making choices about what happens to them during labour. However, not all women are able or want to attend. Many women formalize their decisions before labour by completing a birth plan. This is a written outline of a woman's wishes for her birth. It may cover issues such as what kind of pain relief she would prefer, whether she wants to have electronic fetal monitoring and what position she would like to give birth in.

The use of a birth plan forms part of the National Maternity Records. There are many other alternative versions and examples available to women who have access to the Internet. Some take the form of written lists created by the woman indicating the conditions in which certain interventions will be acceptable and when they will not. Others include a general philosophy of parents' hopes and aspirations for the circumstances in which their baby will be born. Many units use their own particular format to facilitate the birth planning process, often including a tick-box list with some room for specific comments. Although they have the advantage of providing structure to a discussion, they may not reflect the interests of the woman or encourage her to think about what she really wants (Nolan 2001). Kaufman (2008) describes how birth plans can take different forms, such as mind maps and decision trees, to help the woman explore how she feels about birth. The popularity of birth plans has fluctuated, sometimes seen as a hinderance by professionals rather than a tool to enhance woman-centered care. Simkin (2007) argues that birth plans do have a place in contemporary maternity care, that women still want to be heard and that there are practitioners who use them respectfully to enhance the woman's sense of control. *Better Births* (2017:8) states that:

> *Every woman should develop a personalised care plan, with her midwife and other health professionals, which sets out her decisions about her care, reflects her wider health needs and is kept up to date as her pregnancy progresses.*

Activity

Undertake an Internet search for 'birth plans'. Look at some of the examples. Do the requests appear appropriate? Imagine that you were approaching the birth of your first child. What would you consider including in a birth plan? Can you give a rationale for your choices?

Completion of a birth plan provides a useful opportunity for the woman to discuss the available options for the provision of her care (Aragon et al 2013), whether at home or in hospital. Their use may help to enhance communication between midwives and all members of the multi-professional team. Some maternity units have specific policies and targets in relation to the completion of this aspect of the maternity notes, whereas other units do not formally dedicate either time or documentation to this activity. There is evidence that suggests that embedding the birth plan into maternity notes may aid completion, but this does appear to depend on a midwife to facilitate it (Whitford et al 2014). Where the birth plan forms part of care, this requires dedicated time for the midwife and woman to spend time together where the focus of the interaction is not abdominal palpation or blood pressure measurement. However, in reality, it may be combined with an antenatal examination.

Better Births (National Maternity Review 2016) favours a non-prescriptive approach to birth planning to facilitate personalized care. Plotkin (2017) argues that there is no single design that will meet all women's needs.

In ideal circumstances, the midwife would visit the woman at home to discuss the birth plan. One of the main advantages of undertaking this activity in the woman's home is that she is more likely to feel relaxed and able to ask questions in an environment in which she has control. Meeting the woman on her own ground also provides the midwife with much valuable information about the circumstances in which the woman lives and in which she will care for her new baby.

Activity

Find out how birth plans are completed in your locality and how much time the midwife is able to give to this activity.

Implementing birth plans

Irrespective of the form birth plans take, they are not consistently implemented or referred to by midwives, and this can be a source of distress to women (Divall et al 2017). Nolan (2001) makes the point that women are unlikely to make unrealistic, inflexible requests if they have had the opportunity to discuss the birth plan with a midwife. Misconceptions or requests that would be difficult to meet can be discussed before the labour begins. A mutually agreed resolution can usually be found, thus avoiding conflict and disappointment during labour. Some midwives find the use of birth plans 'irritating' due to the higher expectations women may have or if they imply midwives are not going to act in the woman's and baby's 'best interest' (Welsh & Symon 2014). The move toward a personalized care plan, advocated through *Better Births* (National Maternity Review 2016), will mean that more time will need to be given to listening to women and meeting their needs.

The partner's role

Completion of a birth plan is also an opportunity to involve the partner in preparations for the birth. It is argued that there is a strong case for providing information to prospective fathers and including them in antenatal groups to develop skills that will enable them to provide effective support for their partners (Deave & Johnson 2008). A study by Chan and Paterson-Brown (2002) involving 86 fathers and 88 mothers concluded that fathers underestimated how helpful they had been to their partners during labour. Their significant positive contribution to the birth experience when undertaking a supportive role should be emphasized.

A systematic review of caregiver support during labour (provided by either lay people or professionals) demonstrates the continuous presence of a support person in labour increases the chance of normal birth and reduces the likelihood of operative delivery, the need for analgesia and negative feelings after birth (Bohren et al 2017). Evidence also highlights the positive effect of birth doulas for women from socially disadvantaged backgrounds (Gruber et al 2013). When men take on the role of birth partner, however, they can often feel overawed and have difficulty coping with their partner's pain (Kunjappy-Clifton 2008). However, when men have a positive experience of birth, they can benefit both personally and socially through strengthened family relationships (Sweeney & O'Connell 2015).

Activity

How can the midwife encourage birth partners to actively support the laboring woman? What antenatal preparations can they make together to facilitate this process? List 10 ways the partner can participate during the labour.

Place of birth

One of the many advantages of having a home birth is that both the woman and her partner are already familiar with their surroundings. Women who choose to birth their baby in a birth centre or hospital are often coming into an environment that feels strange to them. Wouldn't it be nice if, before we went on holiday, we had a clear idea of the equipment and resources that will be available during our stay? We are not suggesting that coming into a maternity unit to have a baby is like going on holiday, but there are certain useful parallels that can be drawn.

Activity

Access the Birth Place Study and consider what choices are available to women in your locality. Find out how information is provided, and practice how you would provide this information.

Few women have had an opportunity to look around the maternity units available before the birth, accompanied by a midwife or member of the unit who is familiar with the setup. Such a 'guided tour' might have been part of her local antenatal group, where the group arranges to meet at the unit at an agreed date and time. Alternatively, some units have a 'guided tour' perhaps once a week, or there are 'virtual tours' of facilities available on the maternity unit web pages. This enables the maternity unit to be 'seen' at any time of day without disturbing the privacy of the resident women.

Such a tour should ideally include not only a walk around the layout, but also explanations about the function of some of the equipment. For example, she may be introduced to a birth ball or a birthing pool. Women may have heard that an operation theatre is nearby and easily accessible in the event of an emergency, but being shown the physical location may be reassuring.

Having a look around the maternity unit will help women decide what they need to take with them to make their stay more comfortable. Each maternity unit will vary in terms of the facilities it provides. Where possible, the woman should be encouraged to wear her own clothes and retain her own individuality and identity. She will need to take in items of clothing for the baby and to prepare clothes that she wants the baby to come home from the unit in, ready to be brought in on the day they go home. The partner will also need to prepare a small bag including energy-packed snacks, a camera and a list of who to phone when the baby arrives.

Women in special circumstances

When it is expected that a baby is likely to be admitted to the special care baby unit or transitional care ward, then prospective parents are likely to benefit by becoming familiar with the surroundings and meeting a member of staff before the baby is born.

> ### Activity
> In what circumstances might a woman expect her baby to be cared for in a special care baby unit? How does this environment differ from a transitional care facility?

When to call a midwife

Recognizing the onset of labour can be a difficult, particularly for women expecting their first baby. They may be worried about initiating an unnecessary trip to the maternity unit or, conversely, concerned that they might not get to the unit on time. A review of the evidence on self-diagnosis of the onset of active labour (Lauzon & Hodnett 2017) concluded that there was insufficient evidence that giving women specific criteria was any better than general guidelines. Whether the woman is expecting a home or a maternity unit birth, she should be in no doubt about the circumstances in which she should seek professional advice.

Often the local maternity unit, usually the labour ward or 'triage', provides a central role in coordinating the enquiries of women who think they might be in labour or experiencing other problems. Alternatively, some women have direct access to their own community midwife who can assess the situation and provide advice and information for women on her caseload.

The woman should be advised to speak to a midwife if she has:

- Bleeding or abnormal vaginal discharge
- Spontaneous rupture of membranes
- Severe itching
- Severe headache, visual disturbance or epigastric pain
- Reduced fetal movements
- Regular, painful contractions, building in frequency, length and intensity

The midwife should be contacted at the onset of contractions if the woman is booked for elective caesarean section, has a breech presentation, a pre-existing medical condition, a multiple pregnancy, a previous precipitate labour or is not at term.

> **Activity**
>
> Think about the facilities available in your unit for women and their partners. If you were compiling a list of items that a woman might find useful in the maternity unit, what would it include? What would she need to bring in for her baby during the stay? What would you advise partners to bring with them?

Post-term pregnancy

Most labours do not start on the estimated date for the baby' birth, and pregnancy may last up to 42 weeks (NICE 2008). The antenatal guidelines (NICE 2008, 2017) recommend that at 38 weeks pregnant women are informed about the potential risk to the baby of continuing the pregnancy past 42 weeks. It further advises of the need to explain at this time about 'membrane sweeping' – that it increase the chances of labour starting spontaneously and reduces the need for induction of labour. It is also explained what it means to have a membrane sweep and that it may lead to some discomfort and vaginal bleeding. Further information and demonstration of this procedure is in Chapter 7 of book 3, *Labour*.

REFLECTION ON THE TRIGGER SCENARIO

Look back on the trigger scenario.

> *Joanna is now 36 weeks into her pregnancy. She is worried about how her partner, Louis, will support her during labour. Although he has been*

to a couple of classes, there seems to be only one man who says anything, and he has been through the process with another partner. Joanna feels that it is really important to her that Louis takes an active role during the labour. However, she worries that he may be overwhelmed and not feel comfortable with the situation.

Now that you are familiar with issues around preparation for birth, you should have insight into how the scenario relates to the evidence. The jigsaw model will now be used to explore the trigger scenario in more depth.

Effective communication

The midwife needs to communicate effectively with the pregnant woman and her birth partner when she prepares them for the impending birth. She has access to a range of resources to help her do this: one model is the birth plan. Questions that arise from the scenario might include the following: Has Joanna considered completing a birth plan? Has the midwife encouraged her to do this? Has Louis communicated his hopes and fears about the birth to Joanna? Has Joanna talked to Louis about how much she wants him to be involved in the birth? Does he know how important this is to Jo?

Woman-centred care

Attending antenatal classes is one way that prospective parents can get information that enables them to make informed decisions about their care. It also provides an opportunity to explore hopes and fears for birth with their peer group. Questions that arise from the scenario might include the following: Are the classes participant led? Does everyone get the opportunity to voice their individual concerns and aspirations for the birth? How can antenatal classes be facilitated to ensure that they meet the needs of the group rather than the needs of the organization? Are there any opportunities for prospective fathers to get together as a group?

Using best evidence

A range of evidence informs all aspects of maternity care. Accessing appropriate and relevant information is also a challenge for women and their partners. Questions that arise from the scenario might include the following: What are the benefits of attending preparation-for-childbirth groups for the woman and her partner? Is there evidence to support one model of parent education over another? What is the evidence to support Jo's aspirations for the active involvement of her partner during labour and birth?

Professional and legal issues

It is an aspect of a midwife's role to develop an appropriate plan of care for a woman that includes her plans for birth and preparing for parenthood (NMC 2017:6). The midwife can help facilitate a positive birth experience for Joanna and Louis by actively taking Joanna's wishes into consideration. Questions that arise from the scenario might include the following: What organizational factors might prevent the midwife from carrying out Joanna's preferences for labour management? In what circumstances might the midwife need to abandon Joanna's plans for labour? What action should the midwife take if Joanna requested a form of care that the midwife perceives to be unsafe?

Team working

Preparing prospective parents for the birth is predominantly the remit of the midwife. However, there are other key professionals who make an important contribution to this preparation. For example, in some areas, the health visitor, infant feeding advisor, physiotherapist and maternity support worker have a role to play. In addition, the woman may employ the services of a doula. Questions that arise from the scenario might include the following: How might the midwife help Joanna to involve Louis in preparing for the birth? Who might be the most appropriate person to listen to Louis's concerns about the birth?

Clinical dexterity

Midwives work in a range of clinical settings and across the childbirth continuum. They need to keep up to date with all aspects of current practice. Questions that arise from the scenario might include the following: How can community midwives, providing preparation for childbirth groups or individually for women, keep up to date with current practice in their local maternity unit's intrapartum care? What educational resources are available for use in antenatal groups? Are there any education programmes for midwives to help them develop their education skills?

Models of care

Preparation for childbirth groups should take account of the various choices that women make regarding the model of care most appropriate for them. Questions that arise from the scenario might include the following: How might the place of birth affect Louis's confidence to support

Joanna throughout her labour and birth? Is there an opportunity for Louis to become familiar with the birth environment? What model(s) of care would facilitate or hinder the development of trusting relationships between the midwife and her clients?

Safe environment

Sometimes partners feel 'like a spare part' during their partner's labour, lacking the confidence to be an active carer in front of professionals. They need to feel safe to get involved and participate in the process of birth. Questions that arise from the scenario might include the following: What steps can the midwife take to involve Louis in Joanna's care before she comes into hospital? How can he be supported to continue to support Joanna when she comes into the unit? What aspects of the physical labour area environment can be changed to facilitate the active involvement of birth partners?

Promotes health

Women vary in the degree of support they want or expect from their partner. For some, the active support of their partner is felt to be an integral part of the birth experience. Joanna's emotional health is at risk if she has unrealistic expectations of the support that Louis can provide during labour. Questions that arise from the scenario might include the following: How can Joanna and Louis gain a mutual understanding of each other's expectations for the birth? How can the midwife facilitate this?

Further scenarios

The following scenarios enable you to consider how specific situations influence the care the midwife provides. Use the jigsaw model to explore the issues raised in the scenario.

SCENARIO 1

Julie is expecting her second baby. Although her first child is only 3 years old, he was born by elective caesarean, and Julie feels very nervous about the prospect of labour. She has never accessed antenatal groups and is now fearful that she will not be able to cope with her contractions.

Practice point

For some women who have had an elective caesarean for a first birth, the idea of experiencing a labour may be quite daunting. The midwife needs to find out the reason she had an operation the first time round, as this will also guide her choices for subsequent pregnancies. The midwife will require good communication skills to listen the woman's anxieties and help support her.

Further questions specific to Scenario 1 include:
1. Why did Julie have an elective caesarean with her first baby?
2. Was Julie offered antenatal sessions in her first pregnancy?
3. If so, why did she not access them?
4. Was Julie offered antenatal groups this time around?
5. How can Julie be prepared to go into labour with confidence?
6. Has she got a birth partner and, if so, what preparation have they had?

SCENARIO 2

Elizabeth is a school teacher and she has just arrived on the maternity unit with a history of regular contractions for the last 2 hours. After the last contraction, the midwife asks her what she wants to assist her with her pain. Elizabeth replies that she has been practising hypnobirthing and would like to avoid using any pharmacological pain relief, if at all possible.

Practice point

In midwifery practice there is no justification to be judgmental or to label women with a stereotype. Each woman, each labour and each birth are different, and women will make individual choices for their childbirth experience.

Further questions specific to Scenario 2 include:
1. Have you come across pre-conceived ideas from midwives about women who have particular aspirations for birth?
2. Do you have any experience of women using hypnobirthing?
3. What is the evidence to support its use?
4. What actions can you take to ensure that you provide appropriate support to Elizabeth?
5. What action can you take to show respect for Elizabeth's hopes for a drug-free labour?

Conclusion

The unpredictability of the onset and course of labour makes it a difficult event to plan and prepare for. With so many different expectations and experiences to consider, the midwife must assess each woman's situation to help her prepare for the birth. The student midwife has a valuable role to play in helping a woman feel that her specific situation is understood and her hopes respected.

Resources

Best beginnings https://www.bestbeginnings.org.uk/

Fatherhood Institute's research summary: Maternal and Infant health in the perinatal period: the father's role http://www.fatherhoodinstitute.org/uploads/publications/356.pdf

The National Childbirth Trust (NCT) https://www.nct.org.uk/

Birth plans NHS Choices https://www.nhs.uk/conditions/pregnancy-and-baby/pages/birth-plan.aspx

Positive birth movement http://www.positivebirthmovement.org/

RCM Better Births initiative http://betterbirths.rcm.org.uk/

References

Aragon, M., Chhoa, E., Dayan, A., et al., 2013. Perspectives of expectant women and health care providers on birth plans. J. Obstet. Gynaecol. Can. 35 (11), 979–985.

Bohren, M.A., Hofmeyr, G.J., Sakala, C., et al., 2017. Continuous support for women during childbirth. Cochrane Database Syst. Rev. (7), Art. No.: CD003766, doi:10.1002/14651858.CD003766.pub6.

Byrom, S., 2016. Influencing the media – is it a midwife's responsibility? https://mediaandmidwifery.com/2016/08/27/guest-post-sheena-byrom/.

Chan, K., Paterson-Brown, S., 2002. How do fathers feel after accompanying their partners in labour and delivery? J. Obstet. Gynaecol. 22 (1), 11–15.

Cook, K., Loomis, C., 2012. The Impact of Choice and Control on Women's Childbirth Experiences. J. Perinat. Educ. 21 (3), 158–168. doi:10.1891/1058-1243.21.3.158.

Deave, T., Johnson, D., 2008. The transition to parenthood: what does it mean for fathers? J. Adv. Nurs. 63 (6), 626–633.

Divall, B., Spiby, H., Nolan, M., Slade, P., 2017. Plans, Preferences or Going with the Flow: An Online Exploration of Women's Views and Experiences of Birth Plans. Midwifery 54, 29–34.

Fenwick, J., Toohill, J., Gamble, J., et al., 2015. Effects of a midwife psycho-education intervention to reduce childbirth fear on women's birth outcomes and postpartum psychological wellbeing. BMC Pregnancy Childbirth 15, 284. doi:10.1186/s12884-015-0721-y.

Green, J.M., Baston, H.A., 2007. Have Women Become More Willing to Accept Obstetric Interventions and Does This Relate to Mode of Birth? Data from a Prospective Study. Birth 34 (1), 6–13.

Green, J., Baston, H., Easton, S., McCormick, F., 2003. Greater Expectations? Inter-relationships between expectations and experiences of decision making, continuity, choice and control in labour, and psychological outcomes. Summary report. University of Leeds, Mother & Infant Research Unit, Leeds.

Green, J., Coupland, V., Kitzinger, J., 1998. Great expectations. A prospective study of women's expectations and experiences of childbirth. Books for Midwives Press, Hale.

Gruber, K.J., Cupito, S.H., Dobson, C.F., 2013. Impact of Doulas on Healthy Birth Outcomes. J. Perinat. Educ. 22 (1), 49–58. http://doi.org/10.1891/1058-1243.22.1.49.

Haines, H.E., Rubertsson, C., Pallant, J.F., Hildingsson, I., 2012. The influence of women's fear, attitudes and beliefs of childbirth on mode and experience of birth. BMC Pregnancy Childbirth 12, 55. https://doi.org/10.1186/1471-2393-12-55.

Hildingsson, I., 2015. Women's birth expectations, are they fulfilled? Findings from a longitudinal Swedish cohort study. Women Birth 28 (2), e7–e13. doi:10.1016/j.wombi.2015.01.011.

Kaufman, T., 2008. Evolution of the birth plan. MIDIRS - Midwifery Digest 18 (1), 67–70.

Kay, L., Downe, S., Thomson, G., Finlayson, K., 2017. Engaging with birth stories in pregnancy: a hermeneutic phenomenological study of women's experiences across two generations. BMC Pregnancy Childbirth 17, 283. https://doi.org/10.1186/s12884-017-1476-4.

Kunjappy-Clifton, A., 2008. And father came too. A study exploring the role of first time fathers during the birth process and to explore the meaning of the experience for these men: part two. MIDIRS - Midwifery Digest 18 (1), 57–66.

Lauzon, L., Hodnett, E.D., 2017. Antenatal education for self-diagnosis of the onset of active labour at term. Cochrane Database Syst. Rev. (4), Art. No.: CD000935, doi:10.1002/14651858.CD000935.

Lawrence, A., Lewis, L., Hofmeyr, G.J., Styles, C., 2013. Maternal positions and mobility during first stage labour. Cochrane Database Syst. Rev. (8), Art. No.: CD003934, doi:10.1002/14651858.CD003934.pub3.

Luce, A., Cash, M., Hundley, V., et al., 2016. 'Is it realistic?' The portrayal of pregnancy and childbirth in the media. BMC Pregnancy Childbirth 29 (16), 40. doi:10.1186/s12884-016-0827-x.

National Maternity Review, 2016. National Maternity Service Review. Better Births, Improving outcomes of maternity services in England 5 year forward view for the maternity services. DH, London.

National Institute for Health and Care Excellence NICE, 2008, 2017. Antenatal care for uncomplicated pregnancies. https://www.nice.org.uk/guidance/cg62.

National Institute for Health and Care Excellence NICE, 2008. Inducing labour. https://www.nice.org.uk/guidance/cg70.

Nolan, M., 2001. Birth plans. A relic of the past or still a useful tool? Pract. Midwife 4 (5), 38–39.

Nolan, M.L., 2009. Information Giving and Education in Pregnancy: A Review of Qualitative Studies. J. Perinat. Educ. 18 (4), 21–30. http://doi.org/10.1624/105812409X474681.

Nursing and Midwifery Council (NMC), 2017. Standards for competence for registered midwives. https://www.nmc.org.uk/globalassets/sitedocuments/standards/nmc-standards-for-competence-for-registered-midwives.pdf.

Plotkin, L., 2017. Support overdue: Women's experiences of maternity services. The National Federation of Women's Institutes and NCT. https://www

.thewi.org.uk/__data/assets/pdf_file/0009/187965/NCT-nct-WI-report-72dpi.pdf. (Accessed 20 October 2017).

Redshaw, M., Henderson, J., 2015. Safely delivered: a national survey of women's experience of maternity care 2014 Oxford, National Perinatal Epidemiology Unit. https://www.npeu.ox.ac.uk/downloads/files/reports/Safely%20delivered%20 NMS%202014.pdf.

Simkin, P., 2007. Birth plans: after 25 years, women still want to be heard. Birth 34 (1), 49–51.

Sweeney, S., O'Connell, R., 2015. Puts the Magic Back into Life: Fathers' Experience of Planned Home Birth. Women and Birth 28 (2), 148–153.

Sydsjö, G., Blomberg, M., Palmquist, S., et al., 2015. Effects of continuous midwifery labour support for women with severe fear of childbirth. BMC Pregnancy Childbirth 15, 115. doi:10.1186/s12884-015-0548-6.

The Epidural and Position Trial Collaborative Group, 2017. Upright versus lying down position in second stage of labour in nulliparous women with low dose epidural: BUMPES randomised controlled trial. BMJ 359, j4471. http:// dx.doi.org/10.1136/bmj.j4471. (Accessed 20 October 2017).

van Bussel, J.B., Spitz, B., Demyttenaere, K., 2010. Childbirth expectations and experiences and associations with mothers' attitudes to pregnancy, the child and motherhood. J. Reprod. Infant Psychol. 28 (2), 143–160.

Welsh, J.V., Symon, A.G., 2014. Unique and proforma birth plans: a qualitative exploration of midwives' experiences. Midwifery 30 (7), 885–891. doi:10.1016/ j.midw.2014.03.004.

Whitford, H.M., Entwistle, V.A., van Teijlingen, E., et al., 2014. Use of a birth plan within woman-held maternity records: a qualitative study with women and staff in northeast Scotland. Birth 41 (3), 283–289. doi:10.1111/birt.12109.

Wiklund, I., Edman, G., Larsson, C., Andolf, E., 2006. Personality and mode of delivery. Acta Obstet. Gynecol. Scand. 85 (10), 1225–1230.

INDEX

Page numbers followed by '*f*' indicate figures, '*t*' indicate tables, and '*b*' indicate boxes.